Extra
EASY
KETO

Extra EASY KETO

7 Days

{ TO KETOGENIC
WEIGHT LOSS ON
A LOW-CARB DIET }

Stephanie Laska

ST. MARTIN'S
ESSENTIALS
NEW YORK

First published in the United States by
St. Martin's Essentials, an imprint of
St. Martin's Publishing Group

EXTRA EASY KETO. Copyright © 2023 by Stephanie Laska.
All rights reserved. Printed in the United States of America.
For information, address St. Martin's Publishing Group,
120 Broadway, New York, NY 10271.

www.stmartins.com

The Library of Congress Cataloging-in-Publication Data
is available upon request.

ISBN 978-1-250-86169-6 (trade paperback)
ISBN 978-1-250-86170-2 (ebook)

Our books may be purchased in bulk for promotional, educational,
or business use. Please contact your local bookseller or the Macmillan
Corporate and Premium Sales Department at 1-800-221-7945,
extension 5442, or by email at MacmillanSpecialMarkets@macmillan.com.

First Edition: 2023

DIRTY, LAZY, KETO® is a registered trademark of Stephanie Laska and William Laska.
EXTRA EASY KETO™ is a trademark pending of Stephanie Laska and William Laska.

10 9 8 7 6 5 4 3 2 1

To the reader who asked, "Is it too late for me?"
I dedicate this book to you. No matter what your age or
circumstance, we all deserve an honest, fresh start.

Contents

Greetings   *xiii*

INTRODUCTION

Welcome   1

Kinda, Sorta, Keto?   3

You Can Keto   4

Chew on This   5

Keto Questions & Concerns   6

DAY 1: KETOSIS

Bite-Sized Backgrounder   11

Low-Carb Lowdown   13

Kee-Toe Lingo   13

Kindergarten Ketosis   14

Keto Kit & Caboodle   16

Carb Tricks   16

Keto Quiz Checkup   17

Costly Keto Claims   21

Ketosis Confidence   25

Ketosis Checklist   25

Kissable Keto   26

Keto Competency   27

Clear-Cut Keto   28

Crunch-Time Keto   32

Know-It-All Keto Karen   32

Cool (as a Cucumber) Keto Chris   34

Cast of Keto Characters   35

Carefree Keto   35

DAY 2: CARBS

Keep Keto Simple   38

Calibrate Net Carbs   40

Carb Callout   42

Carb Controversy   44

Hooked on Carbs   45

Carb Fight Club   46

Camouflaged Carbs   46

Carb Sharks   47

Carb Divorce   50

Carb Spend Counseling   51

Low-Carb Vegetables   52

Reverse Role Play   52

Common Sense Keto   54

Keto Catastrophe   55

Portion Control Pointers   57

Eyeball Serving Sizes   58

Net Carb Know-How   60

Supersize Serving Size   63

Popsicle Problem   63

Sugar Alcohol Shape-Up   65

Allulose "All-You-Lose"   66

Sugar Shakedown   67

Carbs Gone Wild   69

Carb Crash   70

Carb Chronicles   71

Spoon-Fed Stick-to-Itiveness   72

Day-to-Day Digest   73

Carb Intervention   75

DAY 3: FOOD

One Bite at a Time   78

Considerate Keto   78

FAQs & Observations   92

But It Says "Keto"   93

Cocktails & Caffeine   93

Keto Flu, I Got You!   94

Fast-Forward to Fruit   95

Keto-Friendly Fruit Comparison   96

Fruit Fairness   97

Low-Carb Fruit   98

Vegetable Vulnerability   98

Keto-Friendly Vegetable Comparison   99

Full-Fat Fabulousness   101

High-Fat, Low-Carb Foods   102

Protein Power   102

Protein Pushback   103

High-Protein, Low-Carb Foods   105

Protein Perfection   107

Protein Proof   108

Custom Keto   109

Corner Store Keto   110

DAY 4: MEAL PLANNING

Goof-Proof Plan   113

The Big Three   113

Keto Collaboration   113

Keto Conduct   114

Complete Keto Kit   117

Easy-Peasy Planning   118

Menu Meal Challenge   119

Carb-Counting Clarity   127

Keto Smarter (Not Harder)   128

Low-Carb Lickety-Split   129

Flawed & Fabulous   130

Realistic Workarounds   132

Keto Progress, Not Perfection   133

DAY 5: ROUTINES

Keto Cool Under Pressure   136

Routines Rock (Rules NOT!)   137

Keto Quicksand   138

Captain Keto   139

Keto to Go   152

Routine Wrap-Up   156

DAY 6: PLAY DIRTY

Cut Loose & Keto   158

Questionable Keto   159

That's Not Keto!   160

Keto Candyland   161

Dirty Keto Comfort   164

Carb Crisis   165

Keto Courtroom   166

Dirty Keto Disadvantages   166

"Correct" Keto Sweetener   170

Keto Catch-22   171

Cautionary Keto   173

Keto Conundrum   174

Trick Temptation   175

Advantages of Playing Dirty   177

Keto Coffee Break   178

Keto Copycats   180

Curb Keto Cravings   181

Operation Covert Keto   183

Keto Conviction   185

DAY 7: ALL IN

Keto Karma   187

Keto Crunch Time   188

The DLK Commitment   189

Meal Mix-n-Match   189

Extra Easy Keto Breakfast Ideas   190

Extra Easy Keto Lunch/Dinner Ideas   192

Extra Easy Keto Snack Ideas   194

Extra Easy Keto Dessert Ideas   195

Extra Easy Keto Drink Ideas   197

Bonus Material: 10 *Extra Easy Keto* Starter Recipes   198

Bloopers and Boo-Boos   218

Keto King & Queen   219

Keto Connection   219

Carry On & Keto   220

Keto Countdown   222

Resources   224

Acknowledgments   225

Index   227

Greetings

Dear friend, before you start reading, I want you to know one thing. You are not alone.

I'm Stephanie Laska, and I've stood in your shoes. I've struggled with my weight for my entire life. My earliest childhood memories are related to food, body size, and judgment. The first time I wanted to disappear because of my weight happened in elementary school.

I remember my teacher, Mr. B, ordered everyone to line up by size for recess. I guess he figured it would take us a while (he ducked out to the teacher's lounge for a smoke) though it didn't take me long at all. I knew my exact weight: *eighty-one pounds.*

I was the first person to find my proper place. I can still hear the sound my purple corduroy knickers made as my thighs rubbed together while walking across the classroom. I'm sure no one noticed, but everything at that moment, even my noisy pants, felt absolutely humiliating.

I made my way to the end of the line. I *knew* that was where I belonged. At 81 pounds, I was the tallest and heaviest student in the class.

This was my first memory of thinking something might be wrong with me. My body seemed different from everyone else's. I'm sure there was a time when you felt out of place or stood out for the wrong reasons. For me, that was my moment. Without knowing why I felt deeply ashamed.

My weight was always a "problem." At my heaviest, I weighed close to 300 pounds. That was when I put away the scale (it doesn't work past that number, right?). This was a time in my life that I'd rather forget about. I sweated constantly. I felt uncomfortable in my own skin. Putting on clothes, walking upstairs, and even getting in and out of my car felt like torture.

I wore a size 24, 26, maybe. The end of the line, so to speak. As an adult, I thought, *Well, this is it. Nothing is going to change. This is me.* It wasn't until I was flying to Chicago years later for work that something happened to make me think otherwise.

While the plane prepared for takeoff, I was shocked to find that my seat belt wouldn't clasp. Despite all sorts of creative tugging, no amount of shifting or sucking in helped. I was too mortified to ask the flight attendant for a seat belt extender. Instead, I covered my lap with my suit jacket and pretended to be asleep. My secret was safe. *Or so I told myself.*

My motivation to do something about it didn't entirely materialize that day. The wake-up calls kept coming. I thought about my situation constantly. I knew being heavy wasn't working for me anymore. At the same time, I didn't know what to do about it.

Ever so slowly, I began to search for answers. *What a lonely and miserable experience that was.* The advice people gave me my entire life was contradictory and confusing. It didn't make any sense! Eat this, *not* that. Low-fat, low-calorie? So many rules . . . and nothing seemed to fit. I had already tried those kinds of diets before (and then some). In fact, I felt like an expert. My whole life I'd been on and off diets. I'm sure you can guess the result. *They never ended well.*

I felt confined (and claustrophobic even) when following hard and fast dieting rules. If a particular food was labeled off-limits, it made me want it more. My cravings came wrapped in packages of shame. Though feeling demoralized, I dreamed that someday I could have a healthy relationship with food.

My change in thinking came fast and unexpectedly and caught me entirely off guard. I was at a friend's barbecue, and I noticed her husband had lost a ton of weight. This caught my eye (everyone's, really). Perhaps more interesting than his new size was the heaping plate of tasty-looking food he carried in one hand and a beer in the other.

I became intrigued. It wasn't necessarily because of the chicken (the drink, maybe). It was something else too. *The portion size!* That wasn't the plate of someone who was dieting (or so I thought). He seemed to be going about weight loss in an offbeat way.

According to my friend, he was following his interpretation of the (popular at the time) Atkins diet—picking and choosing which rules to follow. *Who does that?* I wasn't familiar with this kind of confidence. He appeared happy and proud of his choices, not caring what anyone else at the party thought. He was doing what worked for him.

Huh. That got me thinking.

I didn't start following his diet. *No, that would've been too easy!* However, I did become curious. Could I figure out how to lose weight like this too—on my terms?

This moment created a spark. It ignited an itty-bitty fire inside of me. For the first time in many years, I felt hopeful about the possibility of changing my relationship with food and becoming more comfortable in my body.

I started down my own path of self-discovery. The first step? Research. I became a fixture at the library, scouting low-carb diet guides and cookbooks. I felt delighted every time I came across a promising recipe or relatable article. I sifted through boxes of diabetes-focused magazines. Overall, the information seemed conflicting. *Dairy, fruit, brown rice?* Whether or not you should eat these foods seemed contingent on the whims of a petite lady wearing an apron or a sturdy man in a trim lab coat (neither of whom had ever suffered with obesity). Nothing I read provided a solid answer. I was left to figure out weight loss on my own, piecing together tidbits of research that *just made sense*.

Back then, the ketogenic diet, or "keto," was virtually unheard of—mentioned purely in medical circles. A low-carb diet, however, was more familiar. I reflected on the merits of Atkins and South Beach versus the low-fat/low-calorie mindset. I took the good, threw out the bad, and combined it with what I learned about keto since it appealed to me and put theory into practice. Experimentation helped me the most—I ate different types of foods and paid attention to their effects on me. I scrutinized nutrition labels. Right away, I gathered some startling information. Eating foods higher in fat or protein made me feel satisfied for *hours*, while high-carb foods gave me energy for mere minutes (with a backlash of increased cravings, to boot).

Interesting.

Without telling anyone what I was doing, I pressed on. My new way of eating made me feel energized. And yet I didn't feel hungry? To my astonishment, I was losing weight too. I dropped ten pounds the first month. I wasn't convinced. *Could it be a mistake?* I wondered. Silently, not wanting to jinx it, I kept at it.

My metabolic miracle continued, month after month after month, AFTER MONTH. Ten pounds lost became fifty. Fifty grew to one hundred. Over a year and a half, I lost 140 pounds. ONE HUNDRED AND FORTY STINKIN' POUNDS!

It was unbelievable. I couldn't keep my weight loss journey private anymore. Everyone noticed. People I barely knew would walk up to me, demanding to learn more. "HOW did you do it?" I had no clue what to say. There wasn't a name for what I was doing (that I knew of, anyway).

How I responded might seem bewildering. At the time, I said *nothing*. Not a word! I'd clear my throat nervously, turn red in the face, and look around for the nearest exit.

How was I losing weight? Well, it seemed *wrong*. I felt too embarrassed to share even the smallest of details. I wasn't losing weight the traditional way. I didn't count calories, experience hunger pains, or feel deprived (which, in my mind, were the hallmarks of legit "dieting"). I felt like a weight loss bandit. And I didn't feel a twinge of guilt about getting away with my crime!

From an outsider looking in, I didn't necessarily look like someone trying to eat healthier. My quirky eating habits were generally frowned upon, yet they made sense to me. I ate many foods people deemed "bad" (cheese, bacon, sour cream . . .). I regularly enjoyed desserts (sometimes at breakfast). I continued to drink alcohol. I ate when I was moody (sad, happy, or depressed) just like I used to. That part of me didn't change, but I did switch up the foods I ate in those moments. I shopped and cooked in new ways. Creating low-carb recipes helped me to get my "fix." I came to accept my idiosyncrasies.

I let go.

I didn't follow the line of what healthy eating usually looked like, yet to everyone's surprise, I was losing weight. This discrepancy made some people angry. Behaviors like snacking before (or during or after) meals irked people. Eating dessert (even though it was sugar-free) came across as "unfair" (and worthy of comment). Apparently, it didn't jibe with what people thought of dieting. *Show some restraint! Have you no self-control?* The pervading diet culture seems to have everyone brainwashed. I can still hear my grandmother's voice scolding me (at the ripe age of eight) for attempting to order ice cream: "No, no, Stephie. Ladies don't eat dessert. Sweets are *sinful.*"

Even as I grew older, messages about food continued to be confusing and often contradictory. Don't even think of enjoying your food! A hearty appetite MUST be reined in (no matter what's on your plate). *You're so gluttonous.* Starvation and denial were badges of honor in a scale-obsessed society that glamorized the skinny.

I was done playing my part in the charade. *Make it stop!* It was time for me to rewrite the script.

Partway through my journey (I had lost about 50 pounds at the time), I attended a graduation breakfast with extended family at a nice restaurant. I came back from the buffet line holding an overflowing plate of food: scrambled eggs, sausage, strawberries . . . *whipped cream*. I couldn't wait to dive in! The person sitting next to me—a family member, mind you—leaned in to share some "helpful" advice.

"You'd probably lose weight *faster* if you stopped eating so much," he said. The expression on his face was dead serious.

Okay . . . wow. *Did that just happen?* I felt crushed. And humiliated. THIS is why I didn't want to talk about my weight loss. His comment made me so angry! *Where was this jackass when I was 300 pounds and eating Pop-Tarts for breakfast?*

I shut down. Silent, I lowered my gaze and hunched over. I couldn't find the right words (any words!). So, I did nothing. I felt so alone. I just *sat* there, steaming. I didn't even want my strawberries with whipped cream anymore.

I hate talking about my feelings, but they built up to extreme levels during my weight loss journey. I was caught off guard by how volatile I felt. My opinions about food and my reactions to the criticism and disappointment I felt from others—I couldn't keep them inside any longer. I turned to my computer for a solution. It began almost like journaling. Surprisingly, even though I didn't consider myself a writer, per se, expressing my feelings felt cathartic— freeing. Once I started, I couldn't stop. Years of pent-up rants flew onto the page. My thoughts became organized and empowering. Reflecting on my journey helped answer lingering questions I had.

It dawned on me that I'm a bit of a rebel with eating (and life). I avoid doing things the same way as other people. I rarely read directions. *Don't you dare tell me what to do!* It's no wonder my homegrown weight loss strategy appealed to me so much.

Were there other people out there like me? I wanted to know. Would they be interested in a no-holds-barred "keto-ish" lifestyle (without judgment for taking workarounds)?

My desire to find others compelled me to keep going.

On a whim, I made a few attempts to publish what I had written. When it came time to put a label on it, I described my way of eating the best way I knew how: "dirty, lazy, keto." Over time, that description became more official: DIRTY, LAZY, KETO (caps to reflect my excitement). For one, I was playing dirty, breaking all sorts of dieting rules. And at the same time, I lazily did the bare minimum. I created a unique version of the keto diet. In fact, I coined the phrase! No one knew what I was talking about at first.

Kee-toe? Never heard of it. (Shows you how long ago this was!)

She's not a nutritionist or a doctor . . .

Nobody will listen to what she has to say.

Oh, boy. I was in for a long, rough road.

Hearing so many "nos" got me REALLY fired up. I HAD to tell others what I had learned. I discovered, practically by accident, what seemed to be the holy grail for weight loss. Finding another way was life-changing. Nothing would stand in my way from sharing this information. I turned to social media and started a Facebook support group. Sure enough, there were many folks out there, just like me, looking for a sensible solution for how to lose weight. They, too, were tired of following the "rules" of dieting. People not only wanted results but a stress-free and affordable way to achieve them.

Have a sweet tooth? *So what?* Drink Diet Coke. *Who cares!* Some of us are too old to change habits. Maybe WE aren't the ones who need making over. How about the rules about food and dieting change instead?

Trying to eat perfectly all the time is impractical, not to mention demoralizing. Such high standards are difficult to maintain and eventually end in disaster. Failure—over and over again—makes people feel ashamed. They give up! Thank goodness for a better option. It's a keto diet—*with a twist* (*ooh,* that sounds like a cocktail).

DIRTY, LAZY, KETO is not a fad diet. The outcomes are real. The methodology makes sense. It's a solution to the weight loss riddle which has plagued many of us for our entire lives. Is it extreme? Not for me. Maybe not for you either. But that doesn't stop critics from spouting off what they think. Perhaps they feel threatened. Nontraditional ideas question the status quo. It's unnerving to feel that the USDA and current dietary recommendations might have it wrong.

No BREAD? Blasphemous! (Haters rarely attempt to learn more.)

If only they would listen . . . the progress we could make. There are many roads to wellness—none of them inherently right or wrong, just different. When it comes to what we eat, there is room for joyful celebration, for breaking the rules . . . *for dessert.* From multiple covers of *Woman's World* to cooking with Al Roker on NBC's *Today* show, eight books later, I've reached a worldwide audience that agrees. I'm so proud of my part in launching a DIRTY, LAZY, KETO revolution.

Sharing my story has been a journey of soul-searching. Along the way, I realized that it wasn't uniquely about weight loss. My overall health improved. The steps I took weren't complicated; they were extra easy! I found my voice and followed my gut. I learned to have faith in myself.

I want to show you how to do the same.

Introduction

WELCOME

I'm curious about what brought you here. Have you seen firsthand what a ketogenic diet can do? Perhaps a friend, coworker, or family member lost a ton of weight by following a keto diet (and you're dying to figure out HOW). Or have you, yourself, experienced the weight loss wonder of keto . . . *but somehow lost your way?* Wayward dieters, strict keto dropouts, and newbies alike will find solace here. This is a keto, low-carb sanctuary, a rallying point for all.

Welcome to an extra easy way to "do" keto. A method that's equally as potent as the militant, expensive version, but without all the stress and pressure. You don't have to read in the shadows. The secret is out!

If you want to lose weight on a "keto-ish" diet (while having a life), this is the place for you. There are no complicated math equations or *ridonculous* food-related rules to follow here. You won't feel intimidated—not in any way, shape, or form. There's much more flexibility with what foods you can eat here *(making it a lot more fun!).* This lifestyle is doable for everyone. Whether you want to start fresh or need help getting over a hump, I'm here to help you get started.

I may not be a doctor or dietitian, but I speak from personal experience. I lost 140 pounds (half my entire body weight) and have maintained that weight loss for almost a decade. By sharing my story, I've helped thousands *upon thousands* of desperate dieters—worldwide—achieve similar results. I feel so passionate about this way of eating that I've made helping others my life's calling. I'm glad you're here. It's an honor to be your guide on this journey.

DIRTY, LAZY, KETO is not only superior for weight management, but it's sustainable for the long haul. And here's the real kicker—it's surprisingly enjoyable.

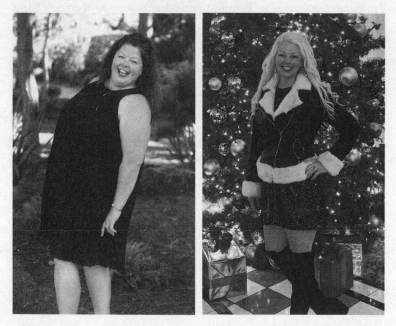

Before and after photos of the author.

KINDA, SORTA, KETO?

A keto diet doesn't have to be executed perfectly to work. There's quite a bit of wiggle room! DIRTY, LAZY, KETO eliminates the unnecessary busy work demanded by fanatics and strips the process down to what matters most. I'll show you which low-carb foods, proteins, and healthy fats will help your body enter the weight loss mecca of ketosis. Equally important, I'll explain *how* and *why* in simple, easy-to-understand terms. All in all, you'll find implementing principles to be fun and manageable. Some say the best part is finding loopholes along the way (this is where "dirty" and "lazy" come in).

> *Strict keto*—meticulous macronutrient and calorie counting with highfalutin standards about the types of food you can eat.
>
> *Dirty keto*—the prerogative to choose foods within your macro goals or limits. Artificial sweeteners, low-carb substitutes, diet soda, alcohol. It's all fair game.
>
> *Lazy keto*—a streamlined tracking system of purposefully counting net carbs (tempered with a sprinkle of common sense).

This "diet" (and I use that term loosely) is like no other. My version of a ketogenic diet is a flexible, real-world approach to eating that might surprise you. There won't be any half-wit rules or impossible standards. You won't find finger-pointing or blaming, either. *Shaming your way to weight loss is a thing of the past.*

I'm going to teach you a kinder and more inclusive method. I believe a little forgiveness translates to confidence and longevity.

People are less likely to drop out if they stumble. The breathing room is so refreshing! It lets you keep your pride. In the long run, engaging in a flexible diet outperforms a rigid approach—*every single time*.

YOU CAN KETO

DIRTY, LAZY, KETO is accessible and uncomplicated. You won't need a calculator or a kitchen scale to make my keto meals. There are no expensive, hard-to-find ingredients or complex ratios for you to figure out. *Everyone* can do this. All you need is a willingness to do your best.

This guide will give you the skill set needed to move forward independently. Freedom, confidence, know-how! That's the differentiator. You'll learn how to accommodate your appetites and preferences within a ketogenic framework. Achieving true success lies in making decisions that are right for *you*. If you can tolerate my sass (and occasional bad joke), I'll support you every step of the way. I promise it will be extra easy.

The reach of DIRTY, LAZY, KETO extends beyond weight loss. You'll look your very best and feel *better* too! This way of eating has astonishing perks for our physical health AND emotional well-being. Commonly reported side effects include:

- feeling energized
- lucid thinking—no brain fog
- less moodiness
- pain-free movement of muscles and joints
- improved digestion

- sound sleep
- stable hormone levels
- breakout-free skin
- no more headaches
- stronger libido
- improved lab reports (standard ranges)
- reversal of chronic health conditions
- bolstered confidence
- a renewed sense of emotional well-being

The effects of the ketogenic diet are life-changing. I treasure the stories readers share with me about how this way of eating has dramatically improved their day-to-day lives. From being able to play on the floor with their grandchildren to no longer needing insulin or a CPAP machine, the underlying message is the same: *they wish they had discovered this way of eating sooner.*

CHEW ON THIS

The medical community is paying attention. Initially hesitant, more and more health care providers are becoming inquisitive about the ketogenic diet and how it can help their patients. "In addition to reducing weight, especially truncal obesity and insulin resistance, low-carb diets also may help improve blood pressure, blood glucose regulation, triglycerides, and HDL cholesterol levels."[1] That's just the beginning. I'm thrilled to learn that the keto diet is being studied for an even broader impact, like treating

1. Wajeed Masood, Pavan Annamaraju, and Kalyan R. Uppaluri, *Ketogenic Diet* (Treasure Island, FL: StatPearls Publishing, 2022).

Alzheimer's disease. Who knows where the research will lead? Keto may very well shape the future of preventative medicine.

"In various studies, the ketogenic diet has shown promising results in a variety of neurological disorders, like epilepsy, dementia, ALS, traumatic brain injury, acne, cancers, and metabolic disorders . . . the ketogenic diet for prevention of type 2 diabetes mellitus or cardiovascular disease may seem premature but is, however, not farfetched."[2]

It's mind-blowing stuff.

KETO QUESTIONS & CONCERNS

I bet you're eager to begin. Is your mind racing? The top ten most frequently asked questions are listed below. I will address each throughout this book. Do any of these issues hit home? (Don't get flustered; I got you.)

1. *Where's the best place to start?*
2. *Which food and drinks are keto-approved?*
3. *How many carbs (or net carbs) do I eat daily?*
4. *Do I count calories too?*
5. *Where's the meal plan and grocery list?*
6. *Explain how these "pee strips" work.*
7. *Can I still do keto if (insert random excuse) . . . ?*
8. *Do vegetable carbs count?*
9. *Is fasting required?*
10. *I want to lose weight* faster! *Show me the tricks?*

---

2. Wajeed Masood, Pavan Annamaraju, and Kalyan R. Uppaluri, *Ketogenic Diet* (Treasure Island, FL: StatPearls Publishing, 2022).

We'll get to the bottom of these topics (and so much more). Here you'll find an accessible keto plan that is efficient, personalized, and actionable. You'll learn *how* to confidently choose the "right" foods and drinks to support weight loss and, equally vital, be able to understand *why*. You won't be going at it alone. I'm going to help you succeed.

Give me seven days. You'll finish the week psyched up and capable of making a meaningful dietary change. Prepare to begin your transformational journey. Expect to stay on target AND achieve your weight loss goals. *Boom!*

DAY 1: KETOSIS

Today we'll start learning the nuts and bolts of DIRTY, LAZY, KETO, a proven way to lose weight and keep it off. You should know from the get-go this is NOT a crash diet. It is a healthy, worthwhile way of eating you can do indefinitely. Ready to roll up your sleeves and get to work? Before you load up a shopping cart on a keto-palooza shopping spree, we've got some strategizing to do.

Starting too fast on a keto diet can backfire. I've seen this time and time again. Folks experience a frenzy of inspiration to start keto RIGHT NOW because they want to lose weight REALLY FAST and make rash decisions. They waste precious time, money, and motivation on fruitless activities that don't pay off.

Keto Booby Traps

Go ahead and chuckle about these widespread mistakes made by wannabe keto dieters. Are any of them unfamiliar? (Kudos to you!) Whatever the case, I won't let you fall into these traps. Throughout this guide, we'll be going into more detail. You'll learn more about each and how to avoid temptation:

- Ordering mysterious "carb blocking" pills or drinks advertised on TikTok.
- Tinkling on pee strips and then FREAKING OUT (*What does this mean!?!*).
- Signing up for a "proven" meal plan (from a dubious stranger on the internet).
- Planning an extended egg fast to jump-start keto weight loss.
- Expecting fraternity-style keto-flu hazing (leg cramps, headache, exhaustion).
- Camping out at a supermarket in hopes of snagging a must-have keto (cardboard) bread.
- Forking over outrageous sums of money for a keto meal-delivery service.

> ⚠️ **Suppress the urge to search for shortcuts, friends. The fast and furious route toward weight loss usually ends up in a disastrous collision (and, ironically, with a return trip to the starting line).**

With no plan or fundamental understanding of how the keto diet works, beginners often blast off with excitement and promptly nosedive. They quit (before really starting), feeling baffled, broke, and bloated. Without ever giving it a real chance, they walk away. *The keto diet doesn't work for me.* I won't let this happen to you!

🔊 **Been there, done that? You're not alone.**

I want to help you avoid unnecessary drama from the get-go. *Start by taking a deep breath.* Put your credit card back in your wallet and find yourself a comfy spot on the couch.

BITE-SIZED BACKGROUNDER

Your first assignment is to understand a ketogenic diet and *why* it works. A teeny tiny physiology lesson. Once you get that, everything else falls into place. (Even I dragged my heels to admit there is value in a science debrief!) Take this step seriously. It can help prevent you from falling down a rabbit hole (rationalizing poor decisions or willingly signing up for keto scams). Spend time reviewing and thoroughly digesting the logical information before you. The goal of Day 1 is to get your mind right. We're going to build a solid foundation before learning anything new.

👣 **Relax and take a load off. Pour yourself a glass of (dry) wine[3] if you'd like (yes, that's allowed) and start studying.**

If you're trying to lose weight, there are limited choices. Between surgery, medication, and exercise, nutrition is the most straightforward option. *Change the foods you eat.* Did those words scare you? Even a whisper about dieting puts most of us in a bad mood. Feeling deprived and hungry all the time is a miserable experience.

---

3. Might I suggest pinot grigio, sauvignon blanc, chardonnay, or pinot noir?

And that's not all. The pounds lost from calorie-restrictive diets are usually temporary (I'm looking at you, Weight Watchers, Jenny Craig, the grapefruit diet). Not being able to stick with it feels demoralizing and shameful. No more, I say. *A keto diet saves the day!*

How it works is so basic. Instead of cutting calories to facilitate weight loss, the keto diet manipulates macronutrients.

Wait . . . what's a macronutrient?

Let me explain (and start from the very beginning). There are three "macronutrients" ("macros" for short) needed by the body to survive and thrive: fat, protein, and carbohydrates. The body can't produce macronutrients on its own—they are consumed in the form of food. Sounds obscure, yet it's pretty clear-cut. On a keto diet, you eat foods that are:

- Higher in fat
- Moderate in protein
- Lower in carbs

How the keto diet helps you lose weight can be summed up in one word—"ketosis"! Ketosis is the effortless way your body burns fat (without a trip to the gym). It happens when the body becomes fueled by fat instead of carbs. *Cool, right? That's my kind of workout.*

Note that you can't "will" or "swill" your way into a metabolic change. Supplements (drinks, powders, pills) have no meaningful potency for controlling ketosis. The body must make the switch on its own. At its very core, the sequence is entirely logical. Ketosis begins when the carbs run out. It only takes a few days. The body is like, *No glucose? No problem. I've got a backup plan.* Then the magic begins.

LOW-CARB LOWDOWN

On a keto diet, your body learns to metabolize food differently than it used to. *Consistently* eating a higher-fat, average-protein, lower-carb diet leads to nutritional ketosis. Just don't let the order of operations confuse you. It's that last part you don't want to miss: *a lower-carb diet*. The body switches gears to ketosis only *after* running out of glucose for energy. Did you catch that? It instinctively hunts for carbs *first*. That, my friends, is ketosis in a nutshell. Mic, drop.

> **After gobbling up the scant amount of carbs in the stomach, the body looks elsewhere for a "bump." In this case, your rump!**

The goal of a keto diet is to get into ketosis. A consistent low-carb diet activates ketosis. Ketosis leads to weight loss.

The mechanics of how the keto diet supports weight loss are straightforward, yet it remains an enigma for most (even doctors!). This way of eating was initially designed to help prevent seizures in people with epilepsy back in the 1940s, before medication was available. Only recently did additional consequences come to light. Fat-burning is just one of the many side effects, though it *certainly* has gained the most attention. It seems EVERYONE these days is talking about keto.

KEE-TOE LINGO

Keto is red-hot. It's become mainstream, baby! Even my local grocery store has added "KETO" callout tags near approved products (in a *willy-nilly* fashion—but they get brownie points for trying).

Ironically, even with so much buzz, most people have no idea what keto, or any of its related jargon, is all about.

"Keto" (short for *ketone* or *ketogenic*) refers to the *keto diet*, a way of eating a diet higher in *fat*, moderate in *protein*, and lower in *carbohydrates*.

Fat: the densest form of energy, providing 9 calories per gram. Examples include vegetable oil, nuts, dairy, avocados, and oily fish.

Protein: a long-chain amino acid, protein takes longer to digest. It has 4 calories per gram and is primarily found in meats, dairy, eggs, legumes, nuts, and seafood.

Carbohydrates: sugars, starches, and fibers that contain 4 calories per gram. Found in packaged or processed foods (from your pantry), and often forgotten about inside fruits, grains, vegetables, and milk products.

Calories: the amount of heat or energy contained in a food. Calories are divided between three main macronutrients: carbohydrate, fat, protein.

KINDERGARTEN KETOSIS

Ketosis is actually a fascinating performance. Eating fewer carbs causes the body's metabolism to change. A reduced carb supply seems to send out a "bat" signal. Alert! ALERT! The carbs are almost *GONE*. After the supply of carbs is metabolized (even the reserves), the body moves on to plan B. It starts to search elsewhere for a hookup. As it turns out, fats (from food and from your body) make a slick alternative.

Who woulda thunk it . . . Fat goes from zero to hero!

> ⚠️ We all know that fat improves the enjoyment of food, but behind the scenes, it does so much more. It provides a condensed form of energy, helps regulate hormone levels, and plays a crucial role in digesting vitamins and minerals. Stores of body fat protect organs and maintain body temperature. We need to stop demonizing this productive macronutrient. Fat is our friend.

Ketogenesis describes the course of action by which fat becomes the new energy source. First, fat is taken to the liver, where it's broken down. As this happens, acids, usually called *ketones* (or *ketone bodies*,[4] *ketoacids*) are produced and released into the blood. Ketones then replace *glucose* (the energy created by carbs) as the body's primary energy source. The exchange is done without a hitch. Ketones are incredibly efficient at doing the job and are readily accepted by the body—no complaints. They fuel all bodily systems—skeletal, muscular, digestive—the whole shebang.

Ketogenesis is a tidy, controlled practice that is totally natural and familiar to the body.[5] It's brought on when a person consistently follows a ketogenic diet. Over time, ketone levels start to build. At a certain point, the body enters a metabolic state of *ketosis*. This is thought to occur when ketone concentrations reach levels below or equal to 0.5mmol/L[6] (which you don't really need to know). *What does mmol/L[7] even mean!?!*

---

4. There are three types of ketone bodies: beta-hydroxybutyrate, acetoacetate, and acetone.

5. As always, when starting any kind of dietary change, be sure to get the approval of your health care provider.

6. Jeff S. Volek and Stephen D. Phinney, *The Art and Science of Low Carbohydrate Living* (Beyond Obesity LLC, 2011).

7. I was trying to be funny, *but in case you really want to know* . . . mmol/L is the international standard

Macronutrient, *shmacronutrient*. Don't overcompli-cate ketosis.

However fascinating to understand, pathophysiology is non-sensical if we don't connect the dots. How will science help you to lose weight? Amen. That's what you want to know. Put the ten-dollar words aside for now. I'll show you the *Extra Easy Keto* way!

KETO KIT & CABOODLE

DIRTY, LAZY, KETO makes ketosis a no-brainer. The principles are easy to follow, and the results are long-lasting. You get to eat decadent, rich-tasting foods (many of which, you'll be delighted to discover, may have been off-limits to you for years). Higher-fat foods like cheese, mayonnaise, nuts, or bacon are now on the table—front and center. You won't be left feeling *hangry* or *angry*.

Emotionally and physically, the variety and amount of food feel satisfying. You continue to enjoy carbs, just less of them. DIRTY, LAZY, KETO teaches you how to adjust the number of macronutrients you eat (and have fun doing it).

CARB TRICKS

On DIRTY, LAZY, KETO, your primary focus needs to be on carbs, not fat. Only by eating fewer carbs can you put ketosis into motion. How you go about eating fewer carbs is up to you. I want to zero in on a popular discipline you may have heard about.

Fasting, or *intermittent fasting (IF),* is simply a planned period

---

unit for measuring how much glucose is concentrated in the blood; specifically, the number of molecules within one liter.

where you intentionally fast or do not eat. Some find this type of structure useful, while others don't see the value—both viewpoints are valid. Let me explain.

You might hear veteran "ketonians" discussing timetables like 16/8, 18/6, 20/4, or 23/1. Each of these numbers refers to fasting hours versus eating hours. Using the first example, in a 16/8, a person might fast from 6:00 P.M. to 10:00 A.M. (16 hours) before their allowable eating window begins from 10:00 A.M. to 6:00 P.M. (8 hours).

The expected fallout of not eating for an extended window is to jump-start ketosis. Physically, there isn't any more food coming in; therefore, the body transitions to fat-burning for energy. Additionally, some tout the emotional upshot of fasting. Anxiety about deciding WHAT to eat finally stops. There are feelings of relief during the break from food. Many find this strategy helps reduce mindless snacking and food intake.

There is no right or wrong way to execute a fast. Resist listening to social media rhetoric and decide for yourself. Is it useful? Maybe, maybe not. But it's not required. From the mild (no eating after dinner) to the extreme (one meal a day—"OMAD"), when you eat is up to you.

> **Fasting, or intermittent fasting (IF), is an optional tool, not a requirement, for losing weight on DIRTY, LAZY, KETO.**

KETO QUIZ CHECKUP

That about covers everything you need to know about K-E-T-O (hey, that rhymes!). Did you process all of that? Just to make sure,

I want to stop and give a pop quiz (I bet THAT got your attention!). There is no need to stress—it's ten questions, guess *true* or *false*. I even provide the correct answers with explanations afterward.

What do you already know—*or think you know*—about ketosis? Sharpen your pencil because we're about to find out.

1. *Ketosis is likely to start once you stop eating foods high in sugar and flour. True or false?*
2. *You must be in ketosis 24/7 to lose and maintain weight loss. True or false?*
3. *Once you fall out of ketosis, it's almost impossible to get back in. True or false?*
4. *Overeating fruit can knock you out of ketosis. True or false?*
5. *Expensive specialty products are a prerequisite for getting into ketosis. True or false?*
6. *"Cheating" on keto can be instantly fixed with exogenous ketones. True or false?*
7. *You can get into ketosis by eating everyday foods from the local grocery store. True or false?*
8. *Ketosis is dangerous. True or false?*
9. *Eating keto-labeled foods from the grocery store is an airtight way to stay in ketosis. True or false?*
10. *The easiest way to get into ketosis (and stay there) is by consistently eating a lower-carb diet. True or false?*

Extra credit: *The only way to tell if you're in ketosis is to pee on those little strips of paper. True or false?*

ANSWER KEY

1. *Ketosis is likely to start once you stop eating foods high in sugar and flour.*

   TRUE—When your body is denied glucose as its energy source (which happens when you stop eating foods high in sugar and wheat flour), it switches to a secondary mechanism, ketosis.

2. *You must be in ketosis 24/7 to lose and maintain weight loss.*

   FALSE—It's a myth that you must *always* stay in ketosis to reap the scale-changing effects of the keto diet. Sure, the more often your body is in ketosis, the higher the likelihood of fat-burning, but be realistic. Will that always be the case? First of all, the body is mysterious. It literally has a mind of its own. Second, everybody makes mistakes! There will likely be moments (knowingly or accidentally) where what you eat knocks you out of ketosis. Think big picture. Don't overreact (but don't delay either). All your hard work, the weight you have lost, will not be wiped out instantly. Focus on returning to the basics, and soon you'll be back on the keto bandwagon.

3. *Once you fall out of ketosis, it's almost impossible to get back in.*

   FALSE—You will re-enter ketosis (usually within 2 to 4 days)[8] once you return to consistently eating a mix

---

8. Cliff J. D. C. Harvey et al., "The Effect of Medium Chain Triglycerides on Time to Nutritional Ketosis and Symptoms of Keto-Induction in Healthy Adults," *Journal of Nutrition and Metabolism* (May 2018).

of higher-fat, moderate-protein, and low-carb foods. Resist the temptation to hunt down a gimmicky short-cut. Instead, take a deep breath. Think about making better food choices starting now.

4. *Overeating fruit can knock you out of ketosis.*

TRUE—Eating too many carbs (even from an organic apple) can flip off the fat-burning switch. Don't take it personally. This is science at work. Too much sugar, even the natural kind, will knock you out of ketosis.

5. *Expensive specialty products are a prerequisite for getting into ketosis.*

FALSE—Ketone drinks, carb blockers, and hocus-pocus supplements are unnecessary for putting your body into ketosis. In fact, I'd go so far as to call these products money-grubbing scams. Do recipes or head-lines sound too good to be true? They probably are. Be skeptical. If it's not your credit card they're after, then beware of ad clicks or data theft. None of these products can expedite or guarantee weight loss.

Hucksters are prolific in keto-land. Promoters take part in multi-level marketing (MLM) pyramid schemes, hoping to get rich preying on your vulnerabilities. They claim their product delivers fast, automatic weight loss . . . *no dietary changes needed!* These snake-oil salesmen use a variety of ploys. They lure you in with clickbait: enticing (fake) before and after photos, catchy TikTok jingles, and wholly fabricated celebrity endorsements ("As Seen on *Shark Tank*," for example—this never happened—a total farce!).

COSTLY KETO CLAIMS

"I lost 50 pounds in six weeks without exercising—message me (or click here) for my meal plan!" (Just wait, next, she'll tell you about the payment plan.)

"Ooh-la-la! Here's the link to my 'Sex in a Pan' chocolate cake recipe." (Clickbait! You'll likely end up on a website riddled with advertisements, the dreamy recipe nowhere to be found.)

"I need inspiration. Show me your before-and-after photos." (Unless you want your identity stolen, be careful about sharing your personal information—including pictures—with strangers.) Scammers will steal your before-and-after images and use them fraudulently to promote their product or program.

Exogenous ketone sales (no, thank you!). These are MLM products promoted by people on payroll.

"Must have" ketone meters, breathalyzers (unnecessary products heavily marketed to you by savvy businesses).

Diet supplements, pills, powders, shakes (watch out . . . it's a hoax—run!).

6. *"Cheating" on keto can be instantly fixed with exogenous ketones.*

    FALSE—There are no shortcuts to ketosis or weight loss, people. Don't be bamboozled! Consuming exogenous ketones hoodwinks you into believing you're bulletproof. Soon after finishing a pricey ketone drink, you can spot ketones in your urine (using those cockamamie pee strips), but *that doesn't mean you're REALLY in ketosis.* You just have expensive pee.

Let me explain. The weight loss part of ketosis happens WAY BEFORE ketones appear in your urine. When the body is fueled by a high-fat, low-carb diet, the kidneys produce ketones during digestion. Ketones are a waste product. The body removes this by-product during urination. As described by Dr. Mike Jones, board certified in obesity medicine (whom you might recognize as the author of the preface for my previous book),[9] "Ketones are the result of fat-burning, NOT the cause."

7. *You can get into ketosis by eating everyday foods from the local grocery store.*

TRUE—Regular food from everyday grocery stores is all you need to get into ketosis and lose weight on a keto diet. The type of ingredients you buy is up to you (organic vegetables, cage-free eggs, line-caught fish, etc.). Strict keto harassment is a thing of the past. No one should be permitted to frown upon your family's budget or values! With DIRTY, LAZY, KETO, there is no pressure. (In case you're wondering, my philosophy is to buy what's on sale.)

Where you shop for groceries won't speed up weight loss. All carbs are metabolized the same way—even when bought from the 99-cent store or the drive-thru.

8. *Ketosis is dangerous.*

FALSE—Ketosis should not be confused with the medical term "ketoacidosis." *Ketosis* leads to fat-burning and weight loss. On the other hand, *ketoacidosis* is a

---

9. Stephanie Laska, *DIRTY, LAZY, KETO (Revised and Expanded): Get Started Losing Weight While Breaking the Rules* (St. Martin's Essentials, 2020).

complication of diabetes that can occur when the body doesn't produce enough insulin, and dangerous levels of acid build up in the bloodstream. That being said, if you're concerned about a medical condition or have specific questions, it's always recommended to consult with your doctor before starting a new diet.

9. *Eating keto-labeled foods from the grocery store is an airtight way to stay in ketosis.*

    FALSE—Manufacturers are now capitalizing on the keto gold rush, promoting keto-branded consumables reminiscent of high-carb favorites: bread, ice cream, cereal, chips, and pizza. So tempting! However, even a cursory glance at the nutrition label might snap your hat back. Keto-advertised foods are often high in calories, scant in serving size, and devoid of quality nutrition. Eating these foods may knock you out of ketosis and even cause weight gain.

 There aren't any free passes for nutrition, folks. Keto convenience foods often lead to a stalling of ketosis or cause a disappointing weight gain.

10. *The easiest way to get into ketosis (and stay there) is by consistently eating a lower-carb diet.*

    TRUE—Consistency is the winning formula. Maintaining a steady diet of low-carb foods helps keep the body in ketosis, a fat-burning state. Low-carb choices, one after another, day after day. Every bite counts.

Extra credit: The only way to tell if you're in ketosis is to pee on those little strips of paper.

FALSE—Ketone levels can be measured symptom- atically or through blood, urine, or breath testing. Urine strips measure the amount of ketones present in urine, but as I'll share in the next section, there are less messy ways to determine whether you're in ketosis. I don't endorse urine strip testing, and here's the official reason why: *they cause people to lose their minds!* Yep. Total crackers.

If you're not aware of the urine test strip procedure, I'll explain how it works. Have you ever tested a swimming pool for chemicals? The directions are similar. A thin plastic test strip passes through a sample (in this case, urine) and is then set aside for a specified time. Processing happens almost immediately; chemical agents on the strip react. You'll notice a change of colors on the test strip if ketones in the urine are detected. Determine concentration levels by comparing the test dipstick against the chromatic scale provided on the packaging.

Deciphering results is cumbersome. False readings occur. Matching up the colors to the key is confusing. The nuance stresses people out (which leads to unnecessary panic). *Am I in ketosis or NOT?! Why isn't the purple DARKER!?* (Friend to friend, please don't post pictures of your urinalysis on social media.)

The whole thing becomes a disaster. People end up second-guessing what they've been eating (not to mention getting themselves all worked up). Stop this obsession before it starts—avoid any testing (urine, breath, blood) for the purposes of a keto diet; these are NOT needed.

KETOSIS CONFIDENCE

Total up your score, then take a moment to reflect. Were there any "aha" moments? The hope was for this exercise to resolve any areas of confusion. Ketosis explains why the keto diet is so advantageous for weight loss, but it doesn't have to feel so darn mysterious.

Ketosis is recognizable once you learn what to expect. Put away the pee strips and breathalyzers. Instead of obsessing over non-specific or ambiguous results, pay attention to changes in your body. This skill set will help you more in the long run. Some symptoms are more glaring than others (the bad breath!), but none of them should cause you any harm. Think of these signals as a heads-up that ketosis is underway.

KETOSIS CHECKLIST

Experiencing one (or more) symptoms should reassure you that you're doing things right.

- weight loss
- lack of hunger
- reduced desire for sweets
- more energy
- clear mental focus
- stable blood sugar levels
- improved skin (fewer breakouts, less eczema)
- reduction in hormonal changes (affecting PCOS, mood swings)
- more restful sleep

- reduced tolerance for alcohol
- increased frequency of urination
- thirst
- occasionally feeling cold
- sharpened sense of smell
- metallic taste or dry mouth
- temporary bad breath (Don't be embarrassed—we'll talk about this next.)

KISSABLE KETO

Halitosis in ketosis? Bad breath is a possible (but short-lived) side effect of entering ketosis.[10] Ketones (b-hydroxybutyrate, aceto-acetate) are associated with an unusual odor, sometimes described as fruity. When ketones are expelled from the body, they can be smelly! Unpleasant side effects will pass with time. Feel free to make tweaks to your diet, like eating a few more carbs, or chewing some sugar-free gum if you experience a metallic taste or dry mouth. *Give it a few days.*

Some fear ketosis will cause their hair to fall out. What a rumor! Sudden hair loss is not an expected side effect of ketosis. So why do some people experience issues with their hair? This phenomenon, also called *telogen effluvium*, is a body's response to stress. Upending the way you eat can shock your system. Thinning hair doesn't happen to everyone who changes their diet, but know that the situation is temporary if it happens to you. Unrelated to diet, hair loss can be symptomatic of an underlying medical condition such as thyroid imbalance, autoimmune disorder, anemia,

---

10. Kathy Musa-Veloso et al., "Breath acetone is a reliable indicator of ketosis in adults consuming ketogenic meals," *The American Journal of Clinical Nutrition* (July 2002).

or PCOS; when in doubt, consult your health care provider for further guidance.

KETO COMPETENCY

Before moving on, stop for a quick knowledge check. There are a lot of "scientific" words and concepts being thrown around, and since we have a variety of learners here, I want to make sure we are all on the same page. Self-assess how you're doing. Can you accurately match each term to the correct definition?

1. *keto diet* _____
2. *ketones* _____
3. *macronutrients* _____
4. *"macros"* _____
5. *fats* _____
6. *proteins* _____
7. *carbohydrates* _____
8. *calories* _____
9. *ketosis* _____
10. *glucose* _____

a. The densest form of energy, providing 9 calories per gram. Examples include oil, nuts, dairy, avocados, and oily fish.
b. Occurs when the body burns ketones from the liver as the main energy source.
c. Short for macronutrients.
d. Blood sugar.
e. A long-chain amino acid, these take longer to digest. Each

gram has 4 calories and it is largely found in meats, dairy, eggs, legumes, nuts, and seafood.

f. Necessary to fuel the body, these come in three forms: fat, protein, and carbohydrate.

g. The amount of heat or energy contained in food (from carbohydrate, fat, or protein).

h. By-product formed in the liver when fat is breaking down (often found in blood or urine).

i. A way of eating that is higher in fat, moderate in protein, and lower in carbohydrates with the goal of achieving ketosis.

j. Sugars, starches, and fibers that contain 4 calories per gram. Found in packaged or manufactured foods (from your pantry), and often forgotten about inside fruits, grains, vegetables, and milk products.

Answer key: 1. i, 2. h, 3. f, 4. c, 5. a, 6. e , 7. j, 8. g, 9. b, 10. d

Now that you have the vocabulary down and have a clear idea of what to expect, you're probably eager to get this party started. *Is there a right or wrong way to get into ketosis? What's the first step?*

CLEAR-CUT KETO

There are two paths to starting a keto diet and getting into ketosis. One is short, straight, and narrow (but laced with treacherous thorns on an extraordinarily steep incline). The other option looks flat and free of debris, but it's suspiciously windy (it might take longer). Eventually, both trails reach the same destination. Which path should you take?

The first is a strict keto diet. It deceptively looks like a straight shot, though you can hardly climb an inch. Draconian keto standards make achieving a weight loss goal (and holding on to it) unnecessarily difficult, if not impossible. Ketosis can only occur when dietary macronutrient goals are *precisely* followed (70% of calories coming from fat, 25% from protein, and 5% from carbohydrates) without any room for error. Exactly 20 grams of "clean" carbohydrates are allowed on any given day—max!

> ⚠️ **Trying to do keto perfectly might last for a day or two, *but then what?* You don't need to make this way of life more complicated than it needs to be.**

A strict keto diet might look like the most expeditious route toward your goal. But realistically, you'll never reach your destination if you can't survive the climb. How can you move forward with useless groceries, calculators, measuring cups, and kitchen scales weighing you down? It's hard to see the path before you, let alone keep macronutrient goals in check.

Militant dieting standards, by design, set you up for failure. Like the preposterous fad diets we've all suffered through (flashback to the grapefruit diet, cabbage soup diet, *cigarette diet!*), a strict keto regimen also makes no sense. It's another style of "do or die" dieting. *No thanks.* Instead, take a closer look at the second option.

It might look like it takes longer, but give it a try anyway. Take a stroll with DIRTY, LAZY, KETO. Enjoy the view! The road to weight loss is flat, uncombative, and accommodates everyone. Sure, there are a few curves, but remain optimistic and you'll soon arrive at your destination. Come to find out, you can kinda sorta follow the same nutritional guidelines of a strict keto diet to reap the rewards of ketosis. *Sneaky, huh.* Weight loss is not the exact science people claim it to be. Work toward the same aim but without stressing yourself out.

- Groceries don't have to be expensive.
- Macronutrient splits don't have to be exact.
- Daily carb counts aren't the same for everybody.
- You don't have to "get all your fats in."
- You're allowed to make mistakes.
- It's okay to enjoy food!
- You can relax while losing weight.

There are many ways to lose weight on a ketogenic diet. You can loosen up the reins and achieve the same outcome. *Hot diggity-dog!* Why choose the more difficult trek (unless you're a glutton for punishment)? An authoritative keto diet will do you no good if it's confusing and overly burdensome to the point that you QUIT.

What's the *best* keto diet? I've got the answer right here. It's the one you can (and will) actually do.

No matter how you attain a state of ketosis, the consequences are identical. Weight loss! Don't be deceived. All keto diets work the same way. One is not more masterful than the other. Review the guiding principles side by side. Which methodology is more reasonable?

Strict Keto Versus DIRTY, LAZY, KETO

Precise calorie and macronutrient formula	Versatile macronutrient model
70% of calories from fat	Higher-fat foods are enjoyed
25% of calories from protein	Protein is regularly eaten
5% of calories from carbohydrates	Carbs are restricted to spur ketosis
Strictly followed	Allows for leeway and personalization
Restricts carb intake to spur ketosis	**Restricts carb intake to spur ketosis**
Strict limit of 20 grams of carbohydrates per day	Flexible range of 20–50 grams of carbohydrates per day
Same rules apply to everyone	Adapts to the individual
Enforces macro consumption ratios	**No rigid macro requirements**
"You must get your fats in."	"Use fat to make healthy food taste better."
"Protein goals are a must."	"Eat some protein at every meal."
"Keep eating until macros are met."	"Use common sense. Stop eating when full."
Time-consuming, complicated math ratios	**Streamlined and simplified carb counting**
Tedious, detailed macronutrient charting	Easy and efficient net carb–focused system
Obsessive fixation on fat, protein, carbs, net carbs, calories—everything!	Quick net carb tracking. One and done.
Advocates counting calories	Counting calories is unnecessary.
Fasting is necessary to spur ketosis	**Fasting is optional to spur ketosis**
Mandates specific intermittent fasting time frames	Believes intermittent fasting, in any format, is a personal choice
Unyielding rules about "allowed" food	**Inclusive, tolerant beliefs about food**
"Clean" eating	"Regular" food
Only organic, natural, whole foods allowed	Choose food you are comfortable with
Nothing processed	No judgment about preservatives or artificial ingredients
Expensive, hard-to-find, specialty ingredients	Affordable, mainstream, familiar foods

CRUNCH-TIME KETO

I understand the allure of wanting to do everything by the book. There's a hope that MORE rules and MORE calorie counting will equate to MORE weight loss—*the sooner, the better!* In reality, this pipe dream falls flat. Making yourself miserable won't help you in the long run. So many rules are likely to backfire. Don't let the hype of "MORE" math mislead you. Rigid diets become overwhelming. Fast. Not being able to maintain the pace makes you feel like quitting. One little snafu? Might as well throw in the towel.

I can't begin to tell you how many folks seek out DIRTY, LAZY, KETO after losing—then gaining—from a strict keto program. The first thing they share is, *I just couldn't keep it up.*

To drive home this point, look at a day in the life of *Know-it-all Keto Karen* versus *Cool Keto Chris.*

KNOW-IT-ALL KETO KAREN

At 0500 hours, a military-style bugle alarm sounds to wake Karen. *On your feet!* There's a lot to do today. Even though her stomach is rumbling, Know-it-all Keto Karen refuses to eat because her predetermined eating window doesn't start for another four hours. Until then, she makes do with a cup of black coffee spiked with MCT oil.[11] Regardless of her apprehension about the MCT oil causing digestive issues (it sure did yesterday), Keto Karen slurps it down—she's famished. Keto Karen is committed to reaching her

---

11. Medium-chain triglyceride (MCT) oil (coconut oil, palm kernel oil) became trendy with the keto community after anecdotal reports circulated that it provides increased energy and aids in leading the body toward ketosis.

fat goals and knows she must start early, come what may. She grins smugly, lips shining with a *perma* lip gloss caused by the pool of coconut oil floating on top of her drink.

Next, Know-it-all Keto Karen lines up her weight loss planning tools like a soldier preparing for battle: Food scale—*check!* Measuring cups—*check!* Graph paper and calculator—double CHECK! She sharpens her pencil and prepares to calculate the macronutrient ratios for today's meals. An hour and a half later, the sun rises; the job is done.

Today, Know-it-all Keto Karen will make every meal entirely from scratch. She has a nine-page shopping list of ingredients to buy for the week (locally sourced organic produce, grass-fed beef, line-caught fish, and cage-free eggs). Shopping and cooking will take up most of the day (and all the cash in her wallet), leaving no time for shenanigans. Better get to the farmers market early—*Do they sell hand-churned butter?* Keto Karen fires off a hasty email, canceling plans with friends. She must buckle down and get serious if she is going to lose weight.

The pattern replays for three days straight. Without a single slipup, Know-it-all Keto Karen pats herself on the back for following the diet *so perfectly*. She brags about her achievement by posting a selfie on Instagram (#eatclean #blessed #ketoforlife) but then lets out a sigh. Though she will admit it to no one, Keto Karen is feeling exhausted. As a "reward," she contemplates taking tomorrow off from her diet. *And maybe the day after that too.*

"I've been so good; I deserve a break! I'll reboot with an egg fast later." (She hopes that eating nothing but eggs for a few days will reverse any weight gain caused by the splurge.)

Know-it-all Keto Karen decides to "start keto again next Monday" (aka never). *No, she didn't!*

COOL (AS A CUCUMBER) KETO CHRIS

After taking the dog for a nice long morning walk, Cool Keto Chris takes a relaxing hot shower and gets set for the day. *I could eat.* For breakfast, she warms up a couple of frozen egg bites in the microwave (broccoli and cheddar, her favorite) to eat during her commute to work. She fills her insulated travel mug with coffee three-quarters of the way, leaving enough space to add something fancy: a splash of sugar-free creamer (a new flavor, pumpkin spice!).

Before heading out the door, Cool Keto Chris takes a moment to think through her calendar. Knowing she has lunch scheduled with the girls at work, she quickly assesses how she plans to spend her carbs today. This is accomplished in a very official way, with hash marks on the back of a napkin.

Lunch will likely be a Cobb salad, and dinner, steak and asparagus on the grill. *Ah, with red wine!* Always thinking ahead, Cool Keto Chris grabs a few snacks to take to the office (celery sticks with peanut butter, a cheese stick, flavored waters, and a Diet Coke). And for the commute? Just in case Chris gets stuck in traffic (and misses dinner), she adds a low-carb protein bar to her bag before heading out the door. Simple.

Chris feels lucky to have discovered a mellow system for losing weight—one that doesn't force her to buy flavorless frozen meals or make boring meal replacement shakes. No endless hours are needed in the kitchen, either. She loves going out to a restaurant with friends, eating the same dinner as her husband, and even having a cocktail.

Slow and steady wins the race! she observes, a relaxed smile on her face. *I can do this forever.*

And so, she does . . .

CAST OF KETO CHARACTERS

Take a moment to reflect on the story. Did you find yourself identifying with one character more than the other? Sure, I threw in a little hyperbole. It's therapeutic to laugh at ourselves, I think. Like many of us, Know-it-all Keto Karen fell into the trap of trying to do everything perfectly. Everyone can relate. (I know I can!) Humor aside, there's a moral to the story here. Holding yourself to such far-reaching standards is not only impractical; it's a recipe for disaster.

You can't game the system. Meaningful change takes time.

Are you thinking about end runs—a three-day egg fast like Keto Karen—hoping to get ahead? (I knew you would catch that.) Let me convince you otherwise. Forcing yourself to eat dozens of eggs is ridiculous (the noxious gas! Sooooo embarrassing.). Will you drop a few pounds? Probably. I'll give you that. But you and I know what happens once you return to your "normal" eating. *The weight comes right back.*

Avoid the madness, people. I've got a better (less stinky) way.

CAREFREE KETO

Let go of extreme measures. Think about *sustainable* weight loss instead. DIRTY, LAZY, KETO is a practical, long-term way of eating that just makes sense.

🔊 **A little breathing room makes a big difference.**

Whew! I think that's enough for today. Understanding ketosis can be a lot to digest. *Ha!* On Day 2, we'll drill down even further. You'll be learning more about the specific macronutrients and how they support weight loss. Lots on the agenda—you better get a restful night's sleep.

See you tomorrow.

Day 1 Marching Orders

1. *Explain the ketogenic diet. How does it work?*
2. *List at least five facts and five falsehoods about ketosis.*
3. *Discuss who is more likely to flourish on a keto diet—Cool Keto Chris or Know-it-all Keto Karen. Why?*

DAY 2: CARBS

Are you anxious to become a card-carrying member of the cool keto club? Joining is hassle-free. Once you see the merit of eating a diet higher in fat, moderate in protein, and lower in carbs, align your food choices to match. The formula is logical, yet people often get LOST. Beginners and keto veterans alike stumble here. The keto basics can feel both overwhelming and confusing. Dieters become so focused on "getting their fats in" or counting grams of protein that they lose sight of what can make or break a ketosis kickstart. Do you know what that is? I'll give you a clue. *It has to do with cutting carbs.*

🔊 **Everything about carbs makes me dizzy. Carbolicious foods are simply intoxicating!**

The word "carb," short for carbohydrate, is neither good nor bad. It's a benign macronutrient unit of measurement that contains 4 calories per gram. Carbs tell you how much sugar, starch, or fiber is inside a given food. When you eat a food rich in carbohydrates, it digests rather quickly. Carbs become a new substance—glucose—a medical term that describes the amount of sugar floating around in your blood.

Eating an abundance of carbs (especially in one sitting) causes glucose to flood your system. Blood sugar levels skyrocket, and you experience a burst of energy. On the flip side, eating foods lower in carbs doesn't cause so much internal hoopla. They have minimal impact on your blood sugar and, therefore, won't give you a false sense of energy.

> ⚠️ **More energy is not better. Consuming more carbs than you need causes a buildup of glucose in the blood. The body stores excess glucose as body fat. *Yikes!***

The effects of eating carbs are predictable. What goes in comes out exactly the same way. Carbohydrate, carb, glucose, (blood) sugar . . . they describe the same thing—energy. For our purposes, from here on out, consider these terms interchangeable. Learning how to manage carb energy (no matter what you call it) will be the focus of Day 2's discussion.

KEEP KETO SIMPLE

I want you to write something down. How about on a sticky note? We're going to start big-picture. Copy down these four steps:

1. *Eat fewer carbs.*
2. *Be choosy about the carbs you eat.*
3. *Stay accurate and consistent.*
4. *Repeat!*

The best plans are simple and easy (extra easy, in fact!). There's no need to overcomplicate weight loss. You just boiled it down to four steps (and the last one shouldn't even count). These principles are the backbone of DIRTY, LAZY, KETO. Post this reminder in a public spot where you can re-read it often. We'll be going into more detail about each step, but these are the highlights.

1. EAT FEWER CARBS.

Limiting carbs is a precursor for launching ketosis. Is there a universal threshold that applies to everyone? Nope. It would be nice if it were that automatic! Unfortunately, this is NOT the case.

> ⚠ **The body won't go into ketosis until all available carbs are exhausted. Don't feed the beast.**

Many keto "experts" draw the line at eating 20 grams of carbs per day (who made them the boss?). In my experience, this ubiquitous limit is inaccurate. Many achieve weight loss with much more than that amount, upwards of 50 grams of carbs per day. Our bodies tolerate varying amounts. That make sense? The amount of carbs you can eat to lose (or maintain) weight varies from person to person. There is no one-size-fits-all rule. Several factors influence your body's carb threshold:

- starting weight (how much you need to lose)
- activity level
- gender
- age
- height

- pre-existing health conditions
- medications

These variables significantly affect metabolism. A person with less to lose, or who is more sedentary, will likely need to eat fewer carbs than a more active person, or someone starting at a much higher weight.

CALIBRATE NET CARBS

To determine how many carbs one can tolerate (to lose or maintain weight loss), you'll need to do a little analysis. Expect some trial and error as you evaluate how your body responds. You might be pleasantly surprised! If you want to start conservatively, begin with 20 grams of *net carbs*[12] per day and see what happens (you can always add more later). Many people can lose weight while eating upwards of 30, 40, or even 50 grams of net carbs per day—in some cases, even more—*hot damn!*

> **I found that giving myself a *range* of carbs to eat helped me stay energized. I lost 140 pounds by enjoying somewhere between 20 and 50 grams of net carbs each day. Having a targeted spread, not an exact number, gave me a little breathing room and allowed real life to happen (and prevented rebellion). For me, having flexibility made the difference.**

---

12. Net carb concept will be explained in more detail later in Day 2.

In any case, be patient as you figure this out. I suggest that you give yourself a whole week before making adjustments. (Not that I want you jumping ahead or anything, but rest assured, sample menus will be provided for various net carb ranges on Day 4.) There is no need to count calories or additional macronutrients during this process. **The DIRTY, LAZY, KETO strategy is to keep it simple and exclusively count net carbs.**

> ⚠ **Make a mental note. Your net carb intake isn't set in stone. It will likely need to be tweaked and adjusted throughout your weight loss journey. Highlight this tip!**

I'll give you a hypothetical situation illustrating how finding your target number (or range) might play out. Say a person starts with eating 20 grams of net carbs per day for seven straight days and ends up losing five pounds.[13] *Ooo-ee!* The following week, a little experiment is done. At 30 grams of net carbs per day for the second week, this person continues to lose weight, dropping an additional three pounds. *Interesting!* For the third week, daily net carbs are padded again, to 40 grams net carbs per day. At this amount, weight loss stalls (there could even be a small gain), though all is not lost.

Conducting this little experiment helped to uncover this person's sweet spot. Can you see how going through these steps helped to reveal valuable information? Following this logic, 20 to 30 grams of net carbs per day facilitated weight loss. Keep in mind the numbers are not universal (I feel the need to say this again).

---

13. Note that the first week on a keto diet usually generates more weight loss compared to later on. Whether due to a loss of water weight or a zealous jump-start, we'll take it!

The rate and the amount of weight lost following a keto diet will differ for everyone.

🔊 **Think of your daily carb spend like cash in your wallet. Once it's gone, it's gone. (No layaway plan, either!)**

2. BE CHOOSY ABOUT THE CARBS YOU EAT.

How will this affect my blood sugar? should guide every decision you make about food. Some foods will come at you like a bat out of hell (donuts, candy, soda, pasta, potatoes, popcorn, rice, corn, even bananas). Others seem to creep up slowly and linger. Weigh the pros and cons of eating diverse carbs and make a plan accordingly.

CARB CALLOUT

A higher-carb food (like a can of non-diet soda) packs a real sucker punch. It's metabolized FAST (before you even know what hits you). Red light! Stop and think twice about proceeding. Because simple carbs digest rapidly, I often refer to them as "fast-burning carbs." These include bread, cereals, sugars, high-sugar fruits, and some starchy vegetables.

Athletes can't get enough of fast-burning carbs. They rely on this immediate energy source for an energetic boost. Bananas, for example, are handed out during marathons. Unless you're running 26.2 miles, exercise caution around these foods.

You don't have to avoid all fast-burning carbs. *Lactose*, the simple, fast-burning carb inside dairy products, is one exception. As you will see on the DIRTY, LAZY, KETO Food Pyramid (coming up next), some low-carb dairy products, like full-fat yogurt, cream, or cottage cheese, can continue to be enjoyed, albeit in small amounts. There's nothing inherently wrong with dairy; think "yellow light." PS: There's another loophole in the fast-burning carb category: low-carb beer and malt liquor fall into this "allowable" category too. You're welcome!

On the opposite end, "slow-burning carbs" are complex carbohydrates that take longer for the body to digest. These are your "green light" foods that let you coast along without feeling hungry. High-fiber fruits, nuts and seeds, and non-starchy vegetables stick around long after you eat them (helping your tummy feel full for longer). This is all thanks to dietary fiber.

Did you know that fiber is a type of carb? This fact surprises many people who falsely assume all carbs are out to get you. Partner up with fibrous carbs and watch the perks pile up. With DIRTY, LAZY, KETO, fiber grams are subtracted from a food's total carb count (which is super cool! Who doesn't love a freebie?).

Similarly, if a food contains any sugar alcohols (more detail about this in just a minute), those grams are also subtracted from the total carbohydrate. Like fiber, the body does not absorb sugar alcohols. They will pass as waste. When calculating net carbs, subtract both. Net carbs reflect the expected impact a food will have on blood sugar.

Choosing what carbs to eat comes with enormous responsibility. It's not that higher-carb foods are evil; they have a foreseeable metabolic effect. No one is punishing you. (I swear!) Too much sugar in the blood eventually leads to weight gain.

 Every year at the holidays, I see the same social media remarks about mashed potatoes: "*I'm going to have*

them. It's not like it's pie!" (Ugh . . . I want to scream, YES, THEY ARE!)

CARB CONTROVERSY

There's a popular saying in keto-land, "If it fits in your macros . . ." (IIFIYM). I interpret this to mean, eat whatever you want as long as you stay within your daily net carb range. While this concept isn't for everyone, for some, having the prerogative to decide for themselves is revolutionary.

Here's a story that drives home this point. I was interviewing a gal for my podcast[14]—an inspiring weight loss transformation story—when our chat took a surprising turn. She started talking about ordering french fries. *Yes, french fries!* (Her remark caught me off guard.) She explained how empowering it makes her feel to order "forbidden" food at a restaurant "while on a *DIET*." After eating five or six fries (with such joy!), her craving is satisfied. Then she boxes up the rest for her dog (that part made me giggle). Here, eating high-carb foods was intentional. It was part of her plan.

Personally, I wouldn't have the discipline to stop myself from eating the entire plate (oh, the appeal of salty fries), but I realize we're all different. I know myself too well. (NONE for me, thanks. I'm a total carb addict!) Where do you fall on the spectrum?

I wonder if you can relate. Can you have a fry or two, then stop? Or, like me, do you lose self-control when tempted with such *carboliciousness*? There is no need to be embarrassed about the latter. There's a whole lot more to the carb story here. It's not your fault.

---

14. DIRTY, LAZY, KETO Podcast by Stephanie Laska.

HOOKED ON CARBS

Carbs are winning a shell game over weight loss. We've been distracted with cutting calories and reducing fat for so long that we've overlooked a discreet villain *hiding in plain sight.* The danger of carbs—as it relates to obesity—has gone downright undetected.

Most of us have been blindsided by their power. (I have never met a baked good that I didn't like!) Carbs can be an alluring temptress—oh, so sweet. Even the USDA thinks carbs are innocent. The dietary guidelines for Americans[15] direct adults to eat 6–8 servings of grains, a whopping 130 grams of carbs *every day.* (That's insane!) No wonder carbs have flown under the radar for so long. They've paraded around as the prom queen of proper health.

Why isn't the government paying more attention? This continues to shock me. Maybe now that the US Centers for Disease Control and Prevention has taken the spotlight in recent headlines, its data concerning obesity will start to gain traction.[16] Take a look at these staggering statistics:

- 74% of adults and 19% of children/adolescents are currently overweight.
- 42% of adults qualify as obese.[17]
- Obesity-related health conditions[18] (which are all preventable!) are among the leading causes of death.

And it's just getting worse . . . the CDC reports the rate of obesity in adults has *tripled* compared to a generation ago (1962 versus

---

15. https://www.dietaryguidelines.gov/

16. https://www.cdc.gov/obesity

17. A body mass index (BMI) of 30 and above is categorized as obese.

18. Type 2 diabetes, heart disease, stroke, even many cancers—all can be avoided.

today). It's shocking. Whatever they have been teaching us about nutrition undoubtedly isn't working. At least for Americans, it seems we've all been duped. This makes me angry and I'm not going to stand for it any longer.

CARB FIGHT CLUB

I'm calling for a do-over with nutrition education. I say we go back to the beginning—time to look at our food options with a fresh set of eyes. To understand which carbs need investigating, we must look beyond the obvious offenders like candy and soda. Tropical fruit, starchy vegetables, bread, even milk—these profiled foods should be at the top of our no-fly list.

We demonize some carbs but not others, making us feel guilty about what we secretly crave. An arbitrary line separates what we should or should not eat. We think it's our fault if we can't follow the "rules." *What a bunch of BS!* Place blame where it belongs. The current nutritional guidelines have created a lose-lose situation. Shoving 6 to 8 servings of grains toward adults every day is like offering a pack of cigarettes to someone trying to quit smoking. Sugar is addictive. It's no wonder we are struggling.

 The first rule of carb fight club is you don't talk about carb fight club. *Admit you know nothing!*

CAMOUFLAGED CARBS

Don't be fooled by appearances. Foods that increase blood sugar often look nutritious. Take breakfast foods, for instance. Bagels, toast, bran cereal . . . I've been told my entire life to eat these foods. They were even recommended to me by my doctor.

Whole grains will help you lose weight, he assured me.

What a crock!

This well-meaning advice did more harm than good. Eating "wholesome" grains like oatmeal caused me to *gain* weight, not lose. I wish I had realized this tidbit a long time ago. It would've saved me a lot of heartache trying to battle the scale (and losing every time). Don't be led astray by semantics. Calling a high-carb food "healthy" is putting lipstick on a pig.

 A word to the wise—be suspicious of carb creeps in disguise!

CARB SHARKS

Don't get conned by these high-carb foods.

- breakfast cereals (grains, bran, granola, corn flakes)
- grains (rice, bread, popcorn)
- muffins (bran, blueberry, pumpkin)
- dried fruit (apricots, dates, raisins)
- tropical fresh fruit (bananas, grapes, pineapple)
- juice (oranges, apples, cranberries)
- fruit smoothies
- granola or granola bars
- low-fat dairy (flavored yogurt, cottage cheese with fruit, cow's milk)
- beans (black, pinto, kidney, refried)

- tortillas (corn, flour)
- starchy vegetables (corn, potatoes, peas, sweet potatoes)

Did any of these high-carb foods surprise you? I expect to hear a resounding "YES." They certainly conned me. I mistakenly thought foods like these were healthy. Granted, I didn't have the best role models. (I spent decades believing french fries counted as a vegetable, for cryin' out loud.) It never occurred to me that something so bland—potatoes, corn, carrots, parsnips (ewwwwwww)—could possibly lead to weight gain. If you're confused, let me set the record straight. Starchy vegetables contain a *bizarre* amount of carbs.

> ⚠️ We carry a lot of emotional baggage about carbs— holidays and culture in particular. Imagine special days without eating a traditional dish—*pasta, rice, beans, naan*? When developing new eating habits, separating *food* from *experience* can become a significant stumbling block.

Take a moment to think about which high-carb foods you might have grief about replacing (or letting go of). Write down your thoughts on paper (old-school style).

I'll go first.

One of my main struggles has always been with popcorn. When I weighed close to 300 pounds, this was my preferred snack. I thought it was harmless (ya know, with all that fiber). I bought "Butter Lovers"–style microwavable bags by the case and polished one off every night while watching TV. When I first started my weight loss journey, I felt remorse for how this habit would have to change. It's embarrassing to admit, but for me, saying goodbye was hard. I missed the experience of mindlessly eating it by the handful.

I came up with a whole bunch of salty substitutes (olives, pickles, bacon, nuts, cheese crisps), but they paled in comparison. (You can't eat a whole bucket of nuts, people.) I couldn't even go to the movies (the smell . . .). I found myself in a tight spot.

I didn't want to abandon my new self-care regimen over a bucket of popcorn. That would be pathetic! I worried if I didn't find a suitable alternative (and soon), I might start feeling resentful. I decided to compromise. Having a small amount (once in a while) was clearly important to me, so I researched my options. I trialed a few brands of lower-carb popcorn (sold in single-portioned bags, score!). It was different from the buttery attraction I was used to— one notch above Styrofoam—but I found it worked in the end.

To this day, going to the movie theater can be hard for me; I have to BOLT past the concession stand. However, knowing I have a smuggled stash of low-carb snacks with me (which now includes salted celery—who knew?), I feel much more confident. Even happy! If I start to miss popcorn (which, to be transparent, happens occasionally), I think about how amazing it feels to sit comfortably in the movie theater chair. THAT feeling? It never gets old.

CARB DIVORCE

Changing your relationship with carbs starts by setting boundaries. You don't have to cut them out of your life completely. Some carbs are beneficial (meat and cheese all day would be uber constipating, after all), but miraculous things start to happen with a reduction. For starters, you'll have more energy. Blood sugar levels stabilize. You'll likely feel less moody or hungry in between meals. There are fewer urges to snack. Your metabolism shifts into high gear (finally!). With your eye on the prize, you become a fat-burning machine.

Emotionally, you might start feeling more in control; this, in turn, helps you become more confident when making food choices. Momentum builds. You become more consistent with the *quantity* and *quality* of your carbs. Suddenly, it hits you. THE MAGIC IS HAPPENING. Your inner transformation has begun. Hallelujah!

The effects of normal, balanced blood sugar reach far beyond weight loss and the bathroom scale. An unforeseen bonus, it reduces our risk of developing cardiovascular disease, type 2 diabetes, hypertension, dementia, and Alzheimer's disease.[19] Impressive, right? When insulin is well-regulated, our whole body and future health reap the rewards.

 Once I finally "got it," my life changed dramatically. Admitting the effects of carbs on my body finally got me to snap out of my carb coma.

---

19. Dylan D. Thomas et al., "Hyperinsulinemia: An Early Indicator of Metabolic Dysfunction," *Journal of the Endocrine Society* (July 2019).

CARB SPEND COUNSELING

Think of your daily allowance of carbs like a budget. How you "spend your carbs" is entirely up to you. But since you're looking for specific guidance, I want to give you sincere advice. You may not like what I'm about to tell you, but here goes anyway. Make vegetable carbs your number one investment. Yes, *vegetables!* It's the biggest bang for your buck. (I bet you didn't see that coming?) As I shared with you earlier, vegetables contain slow-burning carbs that will help you stay fuller for longer (translation: you won't be back roaming the kitchen looking for a snack anytime soon). That's my kind of payout! Heed this advice: *make your carb spend count.*

You don't have to adore vegetables (or even like them all). No matter what the love-hate relationship, eat them anyway. Start with the vegetable(s) you can tolerate the most and go from there. Prepare veggies early and often, with a goal of "just one more" each day. Do what you must to make eating them *bearable*. Pair veggies with fat. Try cooking them in different ways. **Eat plenty of vegetables, and don't hold back**. The carb-smart fiber inside cruciferous vegetables (like broccoli, cabbage, and cauliflower) leaves little leftover space for tempting carby snacks. They will keep you out of the pantry!

> **No one ever became overweight from too many low-carb veggies; let's get real. The carbs inside veggies come from fiber. Faithful fiber is our friend!**

In the battle to manage weight, vegetables give you the upper hand. Do what you must to learn how to eat them. Here are some tips to help you get started.

LOW-CARB VEGETABLES

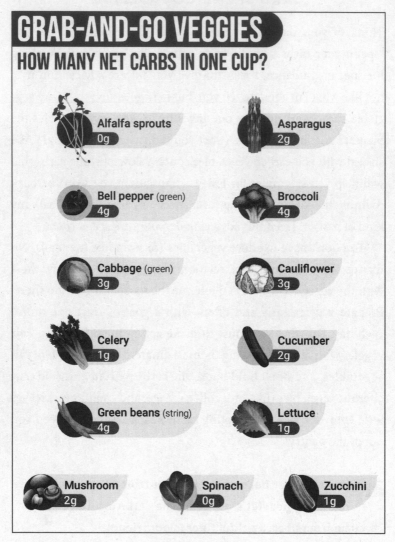

GRAB-AND-GO VEGGIES

HOW MANY NET CARBS IN ONE CUP?

Alfalfa sprouts
0g

Asparagus
2g

Bell pepper (green)
4g

Broccoli
4g

Cabbage (green)
3g

Cauliflower
3g

Celery
1g

Cucumber
2g

Green beans (string)
4g

Lettuce
1g

Mushroom
2g

Spinach
0g

Zucchini
1g

REVERSE ROLE PLAY

Add training wheels: Prepare or serve low-carb veggies with a fat to make them more appealing.

- celery with peanut butter or cream cheese
- raw veggies with ranch dressing dip
- broccoli and cheese
- asparagus with hollandaise sauce
- asparagus wrapped with bacon
- mashed cauliflower (with cream)
- zoodles (zucchini noodles) with pesto or alfredo sauce
- jalapeño poppers
- brussels sprouts sauteed in oil
- stuffed mushrooms (cream cheese)
- creamed spinach
- green beans topped with almond slivers
- roasted radishes (coated in oil)
- fried zucchini patties (shredded vegetables mixed with mozzarella)

Mix it up: Try preparing low-carb vegetables in various ways to change their texture or flavor.

- air-fried (crispy)
- baked (casserole, lasagna)
- blended, mashed, or pureed
- deep-fried
- grilled (shish kebab, barbecued)
- raw (fresh)
- broiled or roasted
- sauteed
- seasoned (salt, pepper, with herbs)
- steamed (pressure cooker, double broiler)
- stir-fried (wok, frying pan)

Sneak 'em in: Whether to fool your brain or strategically make meals more robust, make it a point to add non-starchy vegetables whenever the opportunity arises.

- smoothies (spinach, kale)
- sauces (cauliflower, mushroom)
- pizza base (portabella mushroom, bell pepper, eggplant)
- pizza toppings (bell pepper, tomato, mushroom, olive, jalapeño, broccoli, onion)
- soups/stews (celery, zucchini, cauliflower, mushroom, asparagus, onion)
- sandwiches (lettuce wraps, sprouts, cucumber, spinach, onion, tomato)
- tacos (lettuce, cabbage, tomato, olive, jalapeño, onion)
- taco filling (meat combined with riced cauliflower)
- egg scramble (mushroom, bell pepper, broccoli, tomato, onion)

Like it or not, low-carb vegetables are truly the rocket ship to reach our weight loss goals. Their effects are out of this world (so cheesy, but true!).

COMMON SENSE KETO

Low-carb vegetables aren't the only carbs conducive to weight loss. As you can see from looking at the provided DIRTY, LAZY, KETO Food Pyramid, there are plenty more choices (phew!). Enjoy full-fat dairy, fruit, nuts, and seeds—*within limits*. Why the smaller serving size? Not only are they carb dense, but these foods can be hard to stop eating. Slow your roll. Be mindful of portion control here.

Curious what a day in the life on DIRTY, LAZY, KETO might look like? On the next page is a visual example of how much to eat from each food group.

Keto is not an all-you-can-eat buffet. "No limits" is an urban legend, a falsehood that leads people astray. While this lifestyle feels liberating, there's no such thing as a free lunch.

KETO CATASTROPHE

Case in point, be cautious around the legendary low-carb "fluff" dessert. At first glance, instant pudding/pie filling (sugar-free, fat-free) mixed with heavy whipping cream appears harmless. It tastes delicious and seems to be keto-friendly. *Jackpot!? Don't think so!* Heavy whipping cream is deceptive on a few levels. The nutrition label reveals zero carbs (technically, rounded down from .426) for a tablespoon-size serving. Look what happens when you have more.

For the sake of easy math, imagine using a cup of heavy whipping cream to make this concoction—that's *16 tablespoons*. Unless you plan to eat just *one* tablespoon of fluff (which would be virtually impossible), you've landed in a nutritional minefield. No, we aren't counting fat grams or calories here, but try taking a step back. It's wild! Look how the numbers blow up:

Instant pudding and pie filling mix, chocolate-flavored (sugar-free, fat-free): 42 grams net carbs per 2.1-ounce package (0 grams fat, 180 calories)

Heavy whipping cream: 7 grams net carbs per cup (87 grams fat, 816 calories)

The total damage of eating a cup of fluff: *49 grams net carbs, 87 grams fat, and 996 calories*. Oh my!

DIRTY, LAZY, KETO FOOD PYRAMID

A visual representation of how 20–50g of net carbs per day could be spent

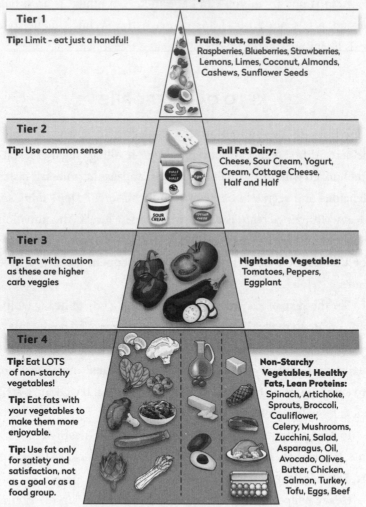

Tier 1

Tip: Limit - eat just a handful!

Fruits, Nuts, and Seeds:
Raspberries, Blueberries, Strawberries, Lemons, Limes, Coconut, Almonds, Cashews, Sunflower Seeds

Tier 2

Tip: Use common sense

Full Fat Dairy:
Cheese, Sour Cream, Yogurt, Cream, Cottage Cheese, Half and Half

Tier 3

Tip: Eat with caution as these are higher carb veggies

Nightshade Vegetables:
Tomatoes, Peppers, Eggplant

Tier 4

Tip: Eat LOTS of non-starchy vegetables!

Tip: Eat fats with your vegetables to make them more enjoyable.

Tip: Use fat only for satiety and satisfaction, not as a goal or as a food group.

Non-Starchy Vegetables, Healthy Fats, Lean Proteins:
Spinach, Artichoke, Sprouts, Broccoli, Cauliflower, Celery, Mushrooms, Zucchini, Salad, Asparagus, Oil, Avocado, Olives, Butter, Chicken, Salmon, Turkey, Tofu, Eggs, Beef

Lean protein, non-starchy vegetables, and healthy fats will help keep you full!

When in doubt, use the DIRTY, LAZY, KETO Food Pyramid on page 56 to reference how best to spend your carbs.

3. STAY ACCURATE AND CONSISTENT.

Enjoy the wide variety of great-tasting DIRTY, LAZY, KETO foods, but at the same time, be responsible. Here's the reality. We are accountable for the foods we choose to eat. Portion sizes are a guiding tool. They keep us honest. If your weight loss stalls or you find yourself feeling hungry between meals, look at the *amount* of what you're eating. Are you overestimating the serving size, or even sadder, shortchanging yourself? You don't have to weigh and measure everything you eat; the eyeballing skill (explained in the provided chart on the next page) can be just as effective.

Now I understand if you struggle in this department. As an overweight person for most of my adult life, my instincts led me astray (they told me to eat an entire box of Triscuits in one sitting). Portion control was a skill I needed to practice. (You should *SEE* my "handful" of nuts!) As such, I developed this cheat sheet for guidance.

PORTION CONTROL POINTERS

In addition to my very official eyeballing technique, I'll share with you some of my own portion-control tips that I have found to be useful.

Trick-or-treat size: When eaten in small amounts, certain low-carb foods have the potential to torment me; nonetheless, I like to have some on hand. In these situations, I don't mind taking on a little extra effort like (1) "spending up" to buy single-serving

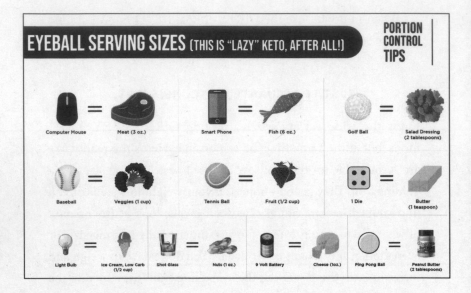

packaging, or (2) creating single-serving units myself (using food storage containers or other sealable packaging) for foods like nuts, olives, or cheese.

Call it a topper: When foods become "unstoppable" as a solo snack, I'll relegate them to "topper" status instead. This strategy works well with berries, nuts, pork rinds, or cheese.

Petite plates: If you're like me and part of the clean plate club, you won't stop eating until every morsel is gone. Serve yourself less from the get-go. Use smaller plates and bowls to deceive your appetite.

Once is enough: Pre-measure frequently used kitchenware now to help monitor serving sizes later. I know that my everyday bowls measure precisely one cup. Whenever I use these dishes, I'm aware of the portion size they hold.

Duplicate measuring sets: Purchase multiple measuring spoons and cups and store them strategically throughout your kitchen to have on hand when needed. If you're like me, these things often get lost or get put back in the wrong places.

> ⚠️ The number of measuring cups I have lying around might seem unnecessary to some, but I find this strategy to be worth the extra effort. No, I'm not weighing or measuring everything I eat. I use them for baking, true, but also to help me monitor portion control of a few hot-button foods. After all, "just winging it" often leads to my eating an entire bag of cheese crisps.

Keep it attached: Leave permanent reminders to help with serving sizes. A shot glass stored next to a container of nuts, to illustrate this idea, will help you accurately scoop out one ounce of nuts.

Adios!: Relocate challenging foods to inconvenient, hard-to-reach locations (the garage, cabinet above the fridge, etc.). If that doesn't help, escalate to plan B. Perhaps only "allow" them when away from the house (like on vacation or at a restaurant). When these measures fail, remove completely from your home for the time being (you can always test the waters again later).

> 📣 I give myself leeway to enjoy certain sugar-free candies *exclusively* when traveling with my family (I'll go overboard with day-to-day access). My kids always seem to want ice cream while on vacation, and as my guilty pleasure, I indulge myself with a once-in-a-while holiday low-carb sweet.

On the go: Ask for restaurant meals to be brought to the table split in half (second portion placed in a to-go container) or order smaller amounts at restaurants (appetizer, side dish, children's meal, a la carte item) in place of an entree.

Coffee house hack: Request the barista to serve your heavy whipping cream or whipped cream separately. Then you can control how much you want to add to your drink.

Preemptive strike: In anticipation of situations beyond one's control, like attending a social event where you don't know the menu, I propose eating low-carb veggies beforehand (to fill up). This strategy physically helps stop you from overeating at the event.

> ⚠️ Sometimes a portion size just isn't fair. Olives contain 1 gram of net carbs per 2 (large) olives or 1 gram net carbs per 5 (medium) olives. *That ain't much!*

NET CARB KNOW-HOW

The most accurate way to figure out the number of net carbs in packaged food is by studying the package's nutrition label. Yes, you can try looking up these details online or through the help of an app, but keep in mind that such information may not be reliable (users may submit the data). Your best bet is to read the label and do the calculations yourself. Keep in mind that nutrition labels vary per country—the provided examples throughout Day 2 are from the United States.

> 👣 When I was a keto newbie, I used a black Sharpie to write the number of net carbs on the packages of every food in my kitchen. This little trick saved me from looking up the same foods over and over, not to mention that it instantly improved my eating choices!

Is a food keto-friendly or not? That's all you need to know. Conservative, strict keto folks waste a lot of time here. They lose sleep poring over the laundry list of ingredients (which is completely unnecessary). Stop scratching your head. Look to the net carb count to give you this information. *Extra Easy Keto* makes the decision-making process a cinch.

Mental math is all it takes. Look at the Nutrition Facts label on any packaged food or nonalcoholic drink to follow along (why most alcoholic beverages do not include this is beyond me). In case you don't feel like walking into the kitchen right now, I'll include one on the next page. Find the **Total Carbohydrate** grams per serving (not the percentage, ignore that). Use this amount as your base. Now subtract any grams of **Dietary Fiber**[20] or **Sugar Alcohol** (if there are any). The result is the number of **net carbs** contained in the listed serving size. *That's it!*

It's interesting to note that in the US, amounts are rounded up or down to the nearest whole number. This is different from products packaged elsewhere that drill down to partial quantities. Who has time to deal with decimals? When in doubt, keep the math simple (numbers you can tabulate in your head). This is DIRTY, *LAZY*, KETO, people.

Practice calculating net carbs using this Chocolate Chip Cookie Dough Protein Bar Nutrition Facts label (yum!). For a one-bar serving, I see it has 22 grams of **Total Carbohydrate**. To calculate **net carbs** for this bar, I'll first subtract any **Dietary Fiber**, listed here as 10 grams, and after that, subtract **Sugar Alcohol**, shown here as Erythritol, 2 grams. The result? 10 grams of net carbs for the entire protein bar.

---

20. Dietary Fiber is the sum of Soluble and Insoluble Fiber.

How to Read a Nutrition Label on Extra Easy Keto

Chocolate Chip Cookie Dough Protein Bar

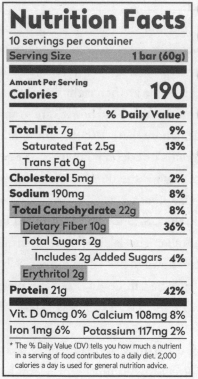

Nutrition Facts

10 servings per container

Serving Size	1 bar (60g)

Amount Per Serving

Calories 190

	% Daily Value*
Total Fat 7g	9%
Saturated Fat 2.5g	13%
Trans Fat 0g	
Cholesterol 5mg	2%
Sodium 190mg	8%
Total Carbohydrate 22g	8%
Dietary Fiber 10g	36%
Total Sugars 2g	
Includes 2g Added Sugars	4%
Erythritol 2g	
Protein 21g	42%

Vit. D 0mcg 0%		Calcium 108mg 8%	
Iron 1mg 6%		Potassium 117mg 2%	

* The % Daily Value (DV) tells you how much a nutrient in a serving of food contributes to a daily diet. 2,000 calories a day is used for general nutrition advice.

1 Notice the serving size. **1 bar**

2 Find the total carbohydrate number. **22**

3 Subtract dietary fiber (if any). **−10**

4 Subtract sugar alcohol (if any). **−2**

5 The result is the **NET CARBS** per serving. **⑩**

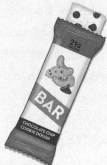

INGREDIENTS: Protein blend (milk protein isolate, whey protein isolate), soluble corn fiber, cashew butter, isomalto-oligosaccharides (vegetable source), unsweetened chocolate, erythritol, water, cocoa butter, natural flavors, sea salt, sunflower lecithin, steviol glycosides (stevia).

CONTAINS: Milk and Cashews

Hopefully, solving that equation didn't cause you to break into a cold sweat. Were you able to arrive at the correct answer without any doubts? Don't be shy. Expect to read over the instructions a few times. It's normal to have a few nagging questions. We will inspect areas where folks often get tripped up.

SUPERSIZE SERVING SIZE

When calculating serving size, the last example was child's play. One protein bar is hard to mess up! It's not always that effortless. Some manufacturers make you jump through a few hoops to determine what constitutes a single portion. *Nothing you can't handle.*

On the next page, you'll find a Nutrition Facts label of a popular frozen treat with a wonky serving size. Take a close look. Are you "supposed to" eat three bars—really? Surprisingly, **Serving size** does not indicate how much you *should* eat. Rather, it reflects how much people *customarily* eat (who these people are, I'm not entirely sure!).

POPSICLE PROBLEM

Here's your task: calculate the number of net carbs in both a serving size (3 bars) and per (1) bar. Go!

Did you come up with the correct answer of 21 grams of net carbs per serving (3 bars), and 7 grams of net carbs per (1) bar? *Well done.* You've officially graduated from the *Extra Easy Keto* Net Carb Academy. Yeah!

For all the overachievers out there wanting a breakdown of each step, here is how I came up with the correct answers. Note

How to Read a Nutrition Label on Extra Easy Keto

Chocolate Popsicle

Nutrition Facts		
4 servings per container		
Serving Size		**3 bars (119g)**
Amount	**Per serving**	**Per bar**
Calories	**120**	**40**
	% DV	**% DV**
Total Fat	2.5g **3%**	1g **1%**
Saturated Fat	1.5g **7%**	0g **0%**
Trans Fat	0g	0g
Cholesterol	less than 5mg **1%**	0mg **0%**
Sodium	130mg **6%**	45mg **2%**
Total Carbohydrate	28g **10%**	9g **3%**
Dietary Fiber	less than 1g **3%**	0g **0%**
Total Sugars	7g	2g
Incl. Added Sugars	0g **0%**	0g **0%**
Sugar Alcohol	7g	2g
Protein	4g	1g
Vitamin D	0mcg **0%**	0mcg **0%**
Calcium	290mg **25%**	100mg **8%**
Iron	0.8mg **4%**	0mg **0%**
Potassium	320mg **6%**	110mg **2%**

* The % Daily Value (DV) tells you how much a nutrient in a serving of food contributes to a daily diet. 2,000 calories a day is used for general nutrition advice.

		3 bars	1 bar
1	Notice the serving size.	*3 bars*	*1 bar*
2	Find the total carbohydrate number.	*28*	*9*
3	Subtract dietary fiber (if any).	*−0*	*−0*
4	Subtract sugar alcohol (if any).	*−7*	*−2*
5	The result is the **NET CARBS** per serving.	*(21)*	*(7)*

INGREDIENTS: NONFAT MILK, MALTODEXTRIN (CORN), SORBITOL, POLYDEXTROSE, COCOA PROCESSED WITH ALKALI LESS THAN 2% OF WHEY, PALM OIL, TRICALCIUM PHOSPHATE, CELLULOSE GEL, MONO AND DICLYCERIDES, CELLULOSE GUM, MASTED BARLEY EXTRACT, SALT, GUAR GUM, ASPARTAME*, POLYSORBATE 80, ACESULFAME POTASSIUM, POLYSORBATE 65, CITRIC ACID, CARRAGEENAN, NATURAL AND ARTIFICIAL FLAVOR, LOCUST BEAN GUM, CARAMEL COLOR
*PHENYLKETONURICS: CONTAINS PHENYLALANINE

there are two columns on the nutrition label: "Per serving" (3 bars) and "Per bar" (which means 1):

Total Carbohydrate: 28g (Per serving), 9g (Per bar)
Subtract Dietary Fiber: 0g (Per serving), 0g (Per bar)
Subtract Sugar Alcohol: 7g (Per serving), 2g (Per bar)
Net carbs: 21g (Per serving), 7g (Per bar)

SUGAR ALCOHOL SHAPE-UP[21]

The body doesn't break down sugar alcohols, so in my book, they don't count. *Sweet!*

Manufacturers may itemize a single sugar alcohol by name, like erythritol. When several sugar alcohols mix, they can lump them all together with the descriptor **Sugar Alcohol**. In the Chocolate Chip Cookie Dough Bar label, the manufacturer identifies the sugar alcohol used: **Erythritol**. (These details come in handy if you experience an unfortunate tolerance issue.)

> ⚠️ **Xylitol is a sugar alcohol that is toxic to dogs. It's often used in sugar-free products like gum, candy, mints, desserts, ice cream, or nut butter, not to mention household products like toothpaste, mouthwash, and medicine. *No sharing and keep out of reach.***

SUGAR ALCOHOLS IN MANUFACTURED PRODUCTS:

- erythritol
- isomalt

21. https://www.accessdata.fda.gov/scripts/InteractiveNutritionFactsLabel/sugar-alcohols.cfm

- lactitol
- maltitol
- mannitol
- hydrogenated starch hydrolysates (HSH)

Suppose the manufacturer chooses *not* to list a sugar alcohol under the carbohydrate section of the label, as is their right (providing no claims about sugar alcohols are made on the packaging). In that case, you'll be forced to inspect the list of **Ingredients**, listed in descending order by physical weight (and scratch your head in wonder about what they're trying to hide).

👣 **Familiarize yourself with what's inside your food and drinks by habitually studying food labels. Ignorance is not bliss!** *Knowledge is power.*

ALLULOSE "ALL-YOU-LOSE"

I won't be able to sleep tonight if I don't include a blurb about Allulose. This relatively new sugar-free sweetener gets a bum rap on the American Nutrition Facts label. It seems to have government officials stumped! Like sugar alcohols, Allulose will not digest by the body. It's a carbohydrate by nature (but the body has no idea what to do with it). How confusing. Allulose becomes lost in nutritional no-man's-land.

How does this affect you? Well, for starters, you'll have a heck of a time trying to figure out the number of net carbs in products that contain Allulose. Since Allulose carbs hide in the Total Carbohydrate category, you'll have no idea how many grams of Allulose to subtract. To illustrate this point, look at the next

Nutrition Facts label. This popular keto cereal advertises 3 grams of net carbs per cup, but exactly how did they come up with this number? Your guess is as good as mine.

Treating Allulose like an everyday carb doesn't seem fair. Allulose is *not* digested by the body, just like the other sugar alcohols, plus it's sugar-free; therefore, in my opinion, it should not count. Here is a unique situation where the FDA has not caught up with emerging science. If the government is listening, can you pretty please amend Nutrition Facts to include Allulose?

Until then, when calculating the net carbs for a product containing Allulose, your only choice is to (blindly) accept the manufacturer's marketing statement about the net carbs on the package.

SUGAR SHAKEDOWN

You might be wondering about **Total Sugars**. *What's the deal?*

Beginners often question if you get to subtract **Total Sugars** from **Total Carbohydrate**. *That's a big no!* Total Sugars is just that—actual sugar. If anything, warning bells should go off. *Ding. DING!* Drop it like it's hot, and don't look back.

Did the thought of eating added sugar scare you? *I hope so!* Eating sugar will spark an endless loop of cravings. It's like an illicit drug. Once you get hooked on sweets again, it becomes almost unbearable to go without. Sugar withdrawal can feel traumatic and emotionally scarring, even. You don't want to *mercilessly* put yourself through that experience again, *do you?* Let go of these high-carb foods and be done with the vicious cycle.

 At least in my experience, "just one bite" often leads to an all-out carb bender.

Keto Cereal (with Allulose)

Nutrition Facts

About 7 servings per container

Serving Size   1 cup (40g)

Amount Per Serving

Calories   **150**

% Daily Value*

Total Fat 6g	**7%**
Saturated Fat 4g	**21%**
Trans Fat 0g	
Polyunsaturated Fat 0g	
Monounsaturated Fat 1g	
Cholesterol 15mg	**5%**
Sodium 75mg	**3%**
Total Carbohydrate 17g	**6%**
Dietary Fiber 5g	**17%**
Soluble Fiber 4g	
Insoluble Fiber 0g	
Total Sugars 1g	
Includes 0g Added Sugars	**0%**
Sugar Alcohol 5g	
Protein 15g	**20%**

Vit. D 0mcg 0%   Potassium 0mg 0%

Iron 0mg 0%   Calcium 230mg 15%

* The % Daily Value (DV) tells you how much a nutrient in a serving of food contributes to a daily diet. 2,000 calories a day is used for general nutrition advice.

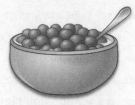

Unlike Dietary Fiber and Sugar Alcohol, Allulose carbs are not identified on a Nutrition Facts label, making it impossible to calculate the number of net carbs.

INGREDIENTS: Milk Protein Concentrate, Erythritol, Allulose, Whey Protein Isolate, Inulin, Palm Kernel Oil, Palm Oil, Soluble Corn Fiber, Canola Oil, Cinnamon, Rice Starch, Soy Lecithin, Natural Flavor, Stevia Extract. Vitamin E (mixed tocopherols) Added to Retain Freshness.

CARBS GONE WILD

Carbs can be your downfall if left unchecked. While it might seem like an innocent idea at the time, eating the occasional high-carb meal or snack can (and probably will) come back to haunt you. The recoil is frightening. Eating too many carbs in one sitting causes your blood sugar to spike—*what a rush*. Your body will convert carbs into high-octane glucose (with a chaser of insulin) PRONTO . . . everything comes alive. *It's electrifying.*

More, more . . . your body seems to shout. When you catch a fever for carbs, you might feel weak, sick, and powerless to stop eating them.

Why does this happen? The biological urge to overeat carbs is probably a throwback to the caveman days when the body was not fed on a consistent and reliable basis. Our forefathers gorged themselves because they did not know when their next meal would be. Call it the Caveman Stockpile Effect (or borrow my hilarious description, Carbs Gone Wild), but cut yourself some slack here. It doesn't matter how you explain it, realize that a carb frenzy is out of your control. The physical pull to overeat carbs is not your fault.

A well-intended snack, say a handful of chips, somehow morphs into a family-sized bag. (HOW does this happen?!) One Chips Ahoy! cookie becomes an entire sleeve. *And it happens fast.*

 When I was hooked on carbs I rarely ever felt full. I would eat a bagel and reach for another ten minutes later. I constantly felt hungry (and ashamed of myself) for wanting to eat so much—and so often! My seeming lack of self-control was embarrassing.

CARB CRASH

Can you guess what happens after a glucose (sugar) rush? *I can!*
Once a carbohydrate buzz wears off, you'll be left tired and grumpy.
To complicate matters, you might start beating yourself up for not
being able to stop yourself. You might even feel hopeless. And so,
self-sabotage begins.

> *Why couldn't I stop myself?*
> *I'll never lose weight!*
> *Might as well eat more carbs.*

Stop yourself from spiraling out of control. Address self-
sabotaging behaviors before they begin. Use these prompts to reflect and take corrective action.

- How do you sabotage your weight loss efforts?
- Pinpoint what triggered you in the past (situations, events, people).
- Imagine a healthier response. What does this look like?
- Make a plan for how to respond to troublesome situations in the future.
- Monitor negative thoughts and practice positive self-talk.
- Take action! Revisit and modify strategies as needed.

Carb "overdoses" can be traumatizing. If the crippling emotions
don't get the best of you, physical cravings will. Plummeting blood
sugar levels cause the body to crave more carbs (for a glucose quick
fix). The frantic, desperate chain of carb-eating events begins all

over again. It becomes a lose-lose situation, no matter what you do. The maniacal response continues with no end in sight.

> 📢 **Say this after me: Carbs beget carbs, beget carbs. Don't let yourself become a carb junkie.**

4. REPEAT!

Only choose foods that your body can handle. And be consistent about it. (Sayonara, Mr. Donut? *She can't be serious.*) It might feel like a big ask (*I just started, Stephanie!*), but I know that you'll soon agree. Saying goodbye to high-carb foods is not punishment. It's liberation! Cutting out high-carb foods is a gift that will *set you free.*

CARB CHRONICLES

Keeping track of your "carb spend" (in a system of your choosing) is especially valuable for beginners and those looking for a fresh start. How else will you know how to make changes? This is your first week. Start strong.

Take pride in your new set of priorities. What you eat, how you feel—all of this matters. Own your truth by documenting the process (the good, the bad, *and* the ugly). Besides providing you with constructive feedback—what is working, what isn't—the very act of monitoring what you eat will help you stay more accountable (to no one else but you).

A system doesn't have to be time-consuming or complicated to be valid. I made a pact with you earlier that there would be no unnecessary busywork, and I stand by that pledge. You're merely counting net carbs with DIRTY, LAZY, KETO (no burdensome macronutrient charting or pie graphs). Down the line, this activity will likely become automatic, but for now, hand-holding is necessary. Make a note of how many net carbs you eat each day at the very minimum. Keep a running tally to prevent going over. *That's it!* Soon this activity will become second nature.

Your system is a personal preference. The format and level of detail are up to you. Some find it necessary to write down specifics (foods, time of day, etc.), while for others, this would be torture (I'm raising my hand). An *Extra Easy Keto* system is best. It needs to be functional, not formal.

SPOON-FED STICK-TO-ITIVENESS

Find what fits and *stick with it*. (I can't emphasize that last part enough.) Many try to skip this step (or half-ass it). Can you predict how this usually turns out? Sloppy. Is that okay with you?[22] My thoughts on this topic have grown more conservative over the years. I've come to appreciate how honesty and tracking tend to go hand-in-hand. Until wishful thinking helps with weight loss, most of us will need a swift kick in the pants and a dependable method for monitoring what they eat. There is no way to sugarcoat this. Accountability entails a little work on your part.

> ⚠ **Without some supervision, most of us end up straying . . . chowing down on Costco samples, and finishing our kids' plates; it never ends. *Every bite counts!***

---

22. I'm not being facetious here. For a slim minority of folks—usually rebels—a loosey-goosey approach (ironically) can yield desired results.

Consider your personality type while forming a plan. Are you more a *chillax*, sticky-note, hashtag kind of a person, like Cool (as a Cucumber) Keto Chris? Or would you fare better with something more exact, perhaps with the help of technology?[23] Either way is fine. Just don't force yourself to do something impractical. There is no sense in relying on an app when your smart device is nowhere to be found (or the extraneous information it provides throws you into a tailspin). Maybe a whiteboard, reproducible worksheet (example provided shortly), or food diary makes more sense. Words are not necessarily needed (you could take photos of what you eat using your phone). Bottom line—think helpful, NOT *homework*.

If posting photos of your nightly dinner on Instagram helps you stay accountable, then do it. On the flip side, though, if seeing other people's food porn makes you feel inadequate, hurry up and log off.

DAY-TO-DAY DIGEST

Assuming you're accurate and consistent with documentation, the payoff is immediate.

Helps you stay focused: It's exciting to see how food choices lead to weight loss.

Can be a reality check (those Costco samples!): Keeping a food log stops you from guessing.

Increases awareness of what and how much you eat: Do you eat

---

23. Popular carb-tracking apps include My Fitness Pal, Carb Manager (the free version), Keto Diet App, and Senza. Keep an ear out—new digital tools pop up all the time.

more (or less) on weekends versus weekdays or at different times of the day? Look for patterns, causes, and effects.

Feedback about what is working (and what is not): The number of net carbs you can eat while in ketosis is not set in stone. Having a record will help you make appropriate adjustments.

DIRTY, LAZY, KETO CARB TRACKER

			TOTAL NET CARBS
MONDAY	breakfast		
	lunch		WATER
	dinner		○○○○○
	snacks		○○○○○
TUESDAY	breakfast		TOTAL NET CARBS
	lunch		WATER
	dinner		○○○○○
	snacks		○○○○○
WEDNESDAY	breakfast		TOTAL NET CARBS
	lunch		WATER
	dinner		○○○○○
	snacks		○○○○○
THURSDAY	breakfast		TOTAL NET CARBS
	lunch		WATER
	dinner		○○○○○
	snacks		○○○○○
FRIDAY	breakfast		TOTAL NET CARBS
	lunch		WATER
	dinner		○○○○○
	snacks		○○○○○
SATURDAY	breakfast		TOTAL NET CARBS
	lunch		WATER
	dinner		○○○○○
	snacks		○○○○○
SUNDAY	breakfast		TOTAL NET CARBS
	lunch		WATER
	dinner		○○○○○
	snacks		○○○○○

NOTES

WEEKLY WEIGH-IN   TODAY'S DATE:

WWW.DIRTYLAZYKETO.COM

The crux of this guide is to teach an undemanding and efficient way to monitor the carbs in your diet.

Exposes nutritional gaps: You might look over a week's worth of notes and find areas for improvement. Did you drink enough water? Maybe you forgot about dairy or aren't eating as many vegetables as you think you are?

Teaches you to trust yourself: You can physically see proof of your new eating habits (cause and effect).

Gives you control of the weight loss process: You have the power to make changes. No one is telling you what to do.

Think of tiny changes like snowflakes. They don't seem to matter until, BAM, you get hit in the head with a giant snowball.

CARB INTERVENTION

All of Day 2 day was devoted to carb education. When you know better, you do better! Feel confident about making calculated decisions. You have the skill set and the background for choosing which carbs to eat and which ones to avoid. And when in doubt? A food diary (of sorts) will provide you with valuable feedback and help you stay focused.

Should you find yourself in a precarious situation (the smell of brownies!), try thinking about the mechanics of how carbs operate to ward off temptation. *Don't laugh—this works!* Beyond taste, it helps to think about how sugar affects the body. How will it make you feel afterward? *So NOT worth it.* I've yet to bite into a cupcake so magnificent it justifies the emotional and physical trauma that goes along with it (and *Lawd* knows I've done the research). The threat is real. Do whatever it takes to make high-carb foods less attractive.

Tomorrow starts the progression from *the why* to *the how*. Stand by! There's even going to be a field trip.

Day 2 Marching Orders

1. *Explain the danger of overeating carbs (until you're blue in the face). Think beyond the scale and contemplate the health implications too.*
2. *Practice calculating net carbs using a variety of nutrition labels.*
3. *Describe how you'll monitor daily net carb spend. Why will this help you?*

DAY 3: FOOD

Here we go! (Sigh.) Another round of crummy and expensive "diet" foods . . .

Did the mention of eating "diet" foods cause you to exhale loudly, thinking life as you know it is over? Let me stop you right there. Cheer up, buttercup. There is no need to squish up your nose in disgust because of the unappetizing foods to come (or bristle about locating specialty ingredients). You won't feel embarrassed, punished, or deprived, either. *There will be none of that here, sir. No, ma'am.*

Day 3 celebrates all the *surprising* foods and drinks you can enjoy on DIRTY, LAZY, KETO. You're going to be thrilled! From cheesy lasagna to low-carb cheesecake, fat-fueled, low-carb foods satisfy hunger, facilitate weight loss, and *taste great*. These keto foods feel familiar. What you're eating doesn't "look like you're on a diet"—this way of eating appeals to everyone.

It helps me to think about what I can have (as opposed to what I can't). Ranch dressing, sour cream, bacon . . . *bring it on!*

ONE BITE AT A TIME

At first, no one feels confident making new food choices on their own. Keto beginners and those seeking a reboot often search out a ready-made meal plan. *I get it!* You want to do everything right. Plus, having all of the work done by an "expert" is comforting. But if you're willing to make a few mistakes at first—getting your hands dirty in the kitchen—the extra effort will soon pay off. I'll provide you with starter meal and snack suggestions (no, I didn't forget dessert!). You'll be off to the races before you know it. Just don't put the cart before the horse (or, in this case, the shopping cart). *Bada-bump!*

CONSIDERATE KETO

Read over the provided grocery list below, pen in hand. Think about each item carefully. Ask yourself, *Which of these foods and drinks do I enjoy eating?* Some might be new to you but sound interesting. Make notes. Take your likes and dislikes into account so you can have a more productive shopping experience later.

> **Pay attention to what foods jump out at you. Any favorites on the list? Draw stars or happy faces next to foods that get you excited. (It doesn't get any more elementary than that.) Add these items to the TOP of your grocery list.**

There are no mandatory foods on DIRTY, LAZY, KETO. Think of the provided grocery list as a keto-friendly directory, like the Yellow Pages (*Uh, oh.* I just dated myself there). By no means are you expected to eat or buy every item shown. No way. You might not like some of these foods, or they may not be in season now, *and that's okay.* Use my suggestions as a starting point.

Do everything in your power to make shopping for nutritious foods pleasurable. A trip to the grocery store should be a worthwhile adventure.

> ⚠️ **Pro tip: Don't waste money buying things you already have. Investigate what's currently in your cabinets and refrigerator before heading to the store. You probably own some of these items and have them stocked in your kitchen.**

DIRTY, LAZY, KETO GROCERY LIST

Drinks

Coffee (black), 0g net carbs per 8 fl. ounces

Diet soda, 0–1g net carb per 8 fl. ounces

Electrolyte-enhanced water,[24] 0g net carbs per 8 fl. ounces

Energy drink (sugar-free or low-carb),[25] 0–3g net carbs per 8 fl. ounces

Flavored drink enhancer (sugar-free), 0–3g net carbs per serving[26]

Hot cocoa mix (note that fat-free hot cocoa mix *has substantially fewer* net carbs than hot cocoa mix with no sugar added!), 4g net carbs per 8-gram serving

---

24. Gatorade Zero, MiO, Powerade Zero Sugar, Propel, Smartwater.

25. Bang, Sugar-free Monster, Sugar-free Red Bull.

26. Serving sizes vary among brands.

Juice (sugar-free grape, sugar-free cranberry),[27] 2g net carbs per 8 fl. ounces

Milk (unsweetened, dairy alternative milk: almond, coconut, cashew, flax, hemp, or soy milk), 0–2g net carbs per cup

Mineral water or flavored water (sugar-free), 0g net carbs per 8 fl. ounces

Protein shake (low-carb, ready-to-drink), 2–3g net carbs per 11.5 fl. ounces

Seltzer water (sugar-free), 0g net carbs per 8 fl. ounces

Soda water (sugar-free), 0g net carbs per 8 fl. ounces

Tea (unsweetened, sugar-free: herbal, black, green), 0g net carbs per 8 fl. ounces

Tonic water (sugar-free), 0g net carbs per 8 fl. ounces

Water (flat), 0g net carbs per 8 fl. ounces

Alcohol

Beer, low-carb (varies by brand), estimated 3–5g net carbs per 12 fl. ounces

Champagne (dry), 1g net carb per 5 fl. ounces

Liquor (unflavored hard alcohol), 0g net carbs per 1.5 fl. ounces

Malt beverages/seltzer, low-carb (varies by brand), estimated 1–5g net carbs per 12 fl. ounces

Wine (dry), 3–4g net carbs per 5 fl. ounces

Dairy (always choose full-fat)

Butter, 0g net carbs per tablespoon

American cheese (processed cheese food), 1–2g net carbs per slice (19–21 grams)

---

27. Ocean Spray (diet juice drink sweetened with sucralose).

Asiago cheese, 0g net carbs per ounce

Blue cheese, 1g net carb per ounce

Brie cheese, 0g net carbs per ounce

Cheddar cheese, 1g net carb per ounce

Cheese (full-fat, block or shredded), 0–1g net carb per ounce

Colby jack cheese, 1g net carb per ounce

Cottage cheese, 4% milkfat, 5g net carbs per ½ cup

Cream cheese, full-fat, 1–2g net carbs per ounce

Eggs, 1g net carb per medium egg

Feta cheese, 1g net carb per ¼ cup

Ghee, 0g net carbs per tablespoon

Goat cheese, 1g net carb per ounce

Gorgonzola cheese, 1g net carb per ounce

Gouda cheese, 0g net carbs per ounce

Gruyère cheese, 0g net carbs per ounce

Half-and-half (full-fat), 1g net carb per 2 tablespoons

Heavy whipping cream, 0g net carbs per tablespoon

Ice cream (low-carb),[28] varies by brand, estimated 0–1g net
    carbs per ½ cup

Milk (unsweetened, dairy alternative milk: almond, coconut,
    cashew, flax, hemp, or soy milk), 0–2g net carbs per cup

Monterey jack cheese, 0g net carbs per ounce

Mozzarella cheese, 1g net carb per ounce

Muenster cheese, 0g net carbs per ounce

Parmesan cheese, 1g net carb per ounce

Pepper jack cheese, 0g net carbs per ounce

Provolone cheese, 1g net carb per ounce

Ricotta cheese (whole milk), 3g net carbs per ¼ cup

---

28. Enlightened, Halo Top, Rebel.

Sour cream (full-fat), 1g net carb per 2 tablespoons

String cheese, 1g net carb per 28-gram serving

Swiss cheese, 0–1g net carbs per ounce

Velveeta cheese, 3g net carbs per ounce

Whipped heavy cream in can (sugar-free), 0g net carbs per 2 tablespoons

Whipped dairy topping in can (regular), 1g net carb per 2 tablespoons

Yogurt (5% milkfat, Greek, strained, plain), varies by brand, estimated 5g net carbs per ¾ cup

Meat, Seafood, & Protein

Bacon (unflavored), 0g net carbs per 2 cooked slices (19 grams)

Beef, 0g net carbs per 3 ounces

Chicken, 0g net carbs per 4 ounces

Chorizo (beef, pork, soy), 4–7g net carbs per 2 ounces

Deli meat (varies by brand), estimated 1g net carb per 2 ounces

Duck, 0g net carb per 4 ounces

Edamame (shelled), 3g net carbs per ½ cup

Eggs, 1g net carb per medium egg

Gyro meat, 5–7g net carbs per 2 ounces

Hot dog (varies by brand), estimated 2g net carbs per link (42 grams)

Jerky (varies by brand), estimated 5–6g net carbs per ounce

Lamb, 0g net carbs per 3 ounces

Lunch meat (varies by brand), estimated 0–2g net carbs per 2 ounces

Meat substitute, formed vegetable protein (varies by brand

and style: crumbles, nuggets, patties), estimated 1–15g net carbs per 3 ounces

Pepperoni, 0g net carbs per 15 slices (28 grams)

Pork, 0g net carb per 3 ounces

Rotisserie chicken, 0g net carb per 4 ounces

Sausage, breakfast (varies by brand), estimated 0–2g net carbs per 2 to 3 links

Seafood (fish, shellfish, shrimp, lobster), 0g net carbs per 3 ounces

Spam, 1g net carb per 2 ounces

Tofu, 0g net carbs per 3 ounces

Turkey, 0g net carbs per 3 ounces

Produce

Alfalfa sprouts, 0g net carbs per cup

Artichoke, 5g net carbs per ½ cup

Arugula, 1g net carb per cup

Asparagus, 2g net carbs per cup

Avocado, 1g net carb per ⅓ medium avocado (50 grams)

Bamboo shoots, 5g net carbs per cup

Bean sprouts, 4g net carbs per cup

Beans (green, wax, Italian), 2g net carbs per ½ cup

Bell pepper (green), 4g net carbs per cup

Bell pepper (red), 12g net carbs per cup

Bell pepper (yellow), 8g net carbs per cup

Blackberries, 6g net carbs per cup

Blueberries, 18g net carbs per cup

Broccoli (fresh), 4g net carbs per cup

Broccoli (frozen), 2g net carbs per cup

Brussels sprouts (fresh), 3g net carbs per ½ cup

Cabbage (bok choy), 1g net carb per cup

Cabbage (green, raw), 3g net carbs per cup

Cauliflower (raw), 3g net carbs per cup

Cauliflower (riced), 2g net carbs per ½ cup

Celery, 1g net carb per cup

Chayote, 4g net carbs per cup

Cherry tomato, 2g net carbs per 3 cherry tomatoes

Chicory greens, 0g net carbs per cup

Chinese cabbage, 1g net carb per cup

Coleslaw mix, 3g net carbs per 1½ cups

Collard greens (cooked), 3g net carbs per cup

Cucumber, 2g net carbs per cup

Daikon (oriental radish, raw), 3g net carbs per cup

Edamame (shelled), 3g net carbs per ½ cup

Eggplant, 2g net carbs per cup

Endive, 0g net carbs per cup

Garlic (fresh), 1g net carb per clove

Ginger (fresh), 0g net carbs per 1 teaspoon or 2g net carbs per 5 slices, 1 inch in diameter (11 grams)

Ginger (dry), 1g net carb per teaspoon

Green bean (string, raw), 4g net carbs per cup

Green onion (raw), 4g net carbs per cup

Heart of palm (canned), 3g net carbs per cup

Herbs, fresh (cilantro, parsley, rosemary, thyme), 0g net carbs per tablespoon

Iceberg lettuce, 1g net carb per cup

Jalapeño (fresh), 1g net carb per ¼ cup

Jicama (raw), 5g net carbs per cup

Kale (cooked), 2g net carbs per ½ cup

Leeks (cooked), 6g net carbs per ½ cup

Lemon, 4g net carbs per medium fruit

Lemon (juice only), 0g net carbs per teaspoon, 1g net carb per tablespoon, 15g net carbs per cup

Lettuce and salad mixes, 1–2g net carbs per 2 cups

Lime, 5g net carbs per medium fruit

Lime (juice only), 0g net carbs per teaspoon, 1g net carb per tablespoon, 19g net carbs per cup

Mushrooms (raw), 2g net carbs per cup

Mustard greens, 1g net carb per cup

Okra, 4g net carbs per cup

Onion (red, yellow, white), 12g net carbs per cup

Pumpkin (fresh, cubed), 7g net carbs per cup

Pepperoncini (sliced), 0–1g net carbs per 12 pieces (30 grams)

Radicchio lettuce, 1g net carb per cup

Radishes, 2g net carbs per cup

Raspberries, 7g net carbs per cup

Rhubarb, 3g net carbs per cup

Romaine lettuce, 1g net carb per cup

Rutabaga (raw), 9g net carbs per cup

Salad greens, 0–1g net carb per 2 cups

Snap peas, 4g net carbs per 1½ cups

Snow peas, 4g net carbs per 1½ cups

Spinach (raw), 0g net carbs per cup

Sprouts (alfalfa), 0g net carbs per cup

Squash (spaghetti), 6g net carbs per cup

Starfruit, 3g net carbs per medium fruit

Strawberries, 8g net carbs per cup

Swiss chard, 2g net carbs per ½ cup

Tomatillos, 1g net carb per ¼ cup

Tomatoes, 5g net carbs per medium tomato

Zucchini, 2–3g net carbs per cup

Baking

Almond flour (super-fine, blanched), 3g net carbs per ¼ cup

Baking powder, 1g net carb per teaspoon

Baking soda, 0g net carbs per teaspoon

Cacao powder (cocoa powder), 100% unsweetened, 1g net carb per tablespoon

Cacao, 85–86% chocolate, 6g net carbs per 2½ pieces (30 grams)

Cacao, 92% chocolate, 6g net carbs per 3 pieces (34 grams)

Carbquik Baking Mix,[29] 2g net carbs per ⅓ cup

Chocolate candy,[30] varies by brand, estimated 1–2g net carbs per 2–5 pieces

Chocolate chips (sugar-free, sweetened with maltitol[31]), 8g net carbs per tablespoon

Chocolate chips (sugar-free, sweetened with monk fruit[32]), 1g net carb per tablespoon

Chocolate chips, dark, 55% cocoa (sugar-free, sweetened with Stevia[33]), 0g net carbs per tablespoon

---

29. Carbquik Baking Mix manufactured by Tova Industries.

30. Russell Stover Assorted Sugar-free Chocolates, Hershey's Sugar-free Chocolate, ChocZero, Lakanto.

31. Hershey's Kitchens Baking Chips.

32. ChocZero, Lakanto, Lily's Sweets.

33. Lily's Sweets.

Chocolate chips, semisweet, 45% cocoa (sugar-free, sweetened with Stevia[34]), 2g net carbs per tablespoon

Chocolate chips, milk chocolate (sugar-free, sweetened with Stevia[35]), 2g net carbs per tablespoon

Chocolate snack bar[36] (low-carb), 2–4g net carbs per 1 (1.4-ounce) bar

Chocolate syrup, sugar-free, 1g net carb per tablespoon

Coconut flour, 4–5g net carbs per ¼ cup

Creole seasoning blend, 0g net carbs per ¼ teaspoon

Gelatin powder (sugar-free), 0g net carbs per ½ cup

Lupin flour, 1g net carb per ¼ cup

Oil (canola, coconut, grapeseed, olive, peanut, sesame, sunflower, safflower, walnut), 0g net carbs per tablespoon

Protein powder[37] (varies by brand), estimated 1–5g net carbs per scoop (30 grams)

Psyllium husk powder, 0g net carb per teaspoon

Pumpkin (canned), 6–8g net carbs per ½ cup

Soy flour, 5g net carbs per ¼ cup

Sugar substitute[38] (Allulose, aspartame, erythritol, sucralose, Stevia, monk fruit), 0g net carbs per packet

TVP[39] (Textured Vegetable Protein), 3g net carbs per ¼ ounce

---

34. Lily's Sweets.

35. Lily's Sweets.

36. Popular brands include Atkins, Quest.

37. Quest brand offers a variety of low-net-carb protein powders.

38. Popular brands include Sugar in the Raw (Allulose), Equal (aspartame), Splenda (sucralose), Truvia (Stevia), Lakanto (monk fruit), Swerve (monk fruit), Sweet'N Low (saccharin). Single packet weight varies by brand.

39. TVP by Bob's Red Mill.

Vanilla (imitation), 0g net carbs per ⅛ teaspoon

Vanilla (pure), 0g net carbs per ⅛ teaspoon

Vital wheat gluten flour, 3g net carbs per ¼ cup

Xanthan gum, 0g net carbs per tablespoon

Nuts and Seeds

Almonds, 3g net carbs per ounce

Brazil nuts, 1g net carb per ounce

Cashews (whole), 8g net carbs per ounce

Chia seeds (black, whole), 0g net carbs per 2 tablespoons

Cocoa roasted almonds, 3g net carbs per packet (17½ grams)

Coconut (unsweetened, shredded), 2g net carbs per 2 tablespoons

Flaxseed (whole), 2g net carbs per 3 tablespoons

Flaxseed meal, 1g net carb per 2 tablespoons

Hazelnuts, 2g net carbs per ounce

Hemp seed hearts (shelled hemp seeds), 0g net carb per 3 tablespoons

Macadamia nuts, 2g net carbs per ounce

Peanuts (roasted, salted), 3g net carbs per ounce

Pecans (halves), 1g net carb per ounce

Pine nuts, 3g net carbs per ounce

Pistachios, 5g net carbs per ½ cup with shells (28g edible portion)

Poppy seeds, 1g net carb per tablespoon

Pumpkin seeds, pepitas (roasted and salted), 2g net carbs per ¼ cup

Sesame seeds, 1g net carb per tablespoon

Sunflower seeds (unshelled), 3g net carbs per ¼ cup

Walnuts (halves and pieces), 2g net carbs per ounce

Sauces & Spices

Au jus gravy mix powder, 1g net carb per ¼ cup prepared
gravy

Barbecue sauce (sugar-free), 2g net carbs per 2 tablespoons

Black pepper (ground), 1g net carb per teaspoon

Bouillon, 0–1g net carbs per half cube or ¼ cup prepared

Chili powder, 1g net carb per teaspoon

Cinnamon (ground or stick), 0g net carb per ⅛ teaspoon

Curry powder, 0g net carbs per ⅛ teaspoon

Everything bagel seasoning *(I admit, an indulgent purchase,
but it packs a punch!),* 0g net carbs per ¼ teaspoon

Garlic (fresh, minced), 1g net carb per teaspoon

Garlic powder, 2g net carbs per teaspoon

Hot sauce (varies by brand), estimated 0–1g net carbs per
teaspoon

Italian seasoning blend, 0g net carbs per ¼ teaspoon

Ketchup (no sugar added), 1g net carb per tablespoon

Marinara sauce[40] (no sugar added), 4g net carbs per ¼ cup

Mayonnaise (full-fat), 0g net carbs per tablespoon

Mustard (yellow, spicy, or dry), 0g net carbs per teaspoon

Onion powder, 2g net carbs per teaspoon

Pancake syrup (sugar-free), 0g net carbs per 2 tablespoons

Ranch powder mix, 1g net carb per ½ teaspoon

Salad dressing (blue cheese, Caesar, creamy Italian, ranch),
1–3g net carbs per 2 tablespoons

Salt, 0g net carbs per ⅛ teaspoon

Sriracha sauce, 1g net carb per tablespoon

Soy sauce, 1g net carb per tablespoon

---

40. Hunt's 100% Natural Tomato Sauce, Hunt's Pasta Sauce (No Added Sugar), Rao's Homemade.

Syrup (flavored, sugar-free), 0–1g net carb per 2 tablespoons

Taco powder seasoning, 3g net carbs per 2 teaspoons

Turmeric powder, 0g net carbs per ⅛ teaspoon

Vinegar (apple cider vinegar, white), 0g net carbs per tablespoon

Worcestershire sauce, 1g net carb per teaspoon

Cans, Bottles, & Jars

Alfredo sauce, 4g net carbs per ¼ cup

Barbeque sauce (sugar-free), 2g net carbs per 2 tablespoons

Broth (canned), 1g net carb per cup

Chicken (canned), 0g net carbs per 2 ounces

Chiles (green, diced), 6g net carbs per ½ cup

Clams (canned), 2–3g net carbs per 3 ounces

Coconut milk (canned, unsweetened, 12–14% fat), 1g net
carb per 2.7 fl. ounces or ⅓ cup

Crab meat[41] (real, canned), 2g net carbs per 4.25 ounce

Enchilada sauce (green or red), 4g net carbs per ¼ cup

Gravy (canned; turkey, chicken, beef), varies by brand, estimated 3–4g net carbs per ¼ cup

Jam, jelly, and preserves (sugar-free), 3–5g net carbs per
tablespoon

Lemon juice (100% juice from concentrate), 0g net carb
per teaspoon, 1g net carb per tablespoon, 15g net carbs
per cup

Lime juice (100% juice from concentrate), 0g net carb per
teaspoon, 1g net carb per tablespoon, 19g net carbs per
cup

---

41. Avoid imitation crab meat which contains added sugar.

Nut butter (no sugar added), 3–6g net carbs per 2 tablespoons

Olives (black, green), 1g net carb per 2 large olives, 1g net
carb per 5 medium olives

Pasta sauce[42] (no sugar added), 4g net carbs per ¼ cup

Peanut butter, 6g net carbs per 2 tablespoons

Pesto, 1–5g net carbs per ¼ cup

Pickles[43] (dill), 1–2g net carbs per spear (1-ounce)

Pumpkin (100% pure, canned), 6–8g net carbs per ½ cup

Salmon (canned), 0g net carbs per 5 ounces

Sardines (canned in oil), 0g net carbs per ¼ cup

Tuna (canned in oil), 0g net carbs per 2 ounces

Vienna sausage, 1g net carb per 60-gram serving

Miscellaneous

Chocolate frozen dessert bar[44] (sugar-free or no sugar
added), varies by brand, estimated 2–6g net carbs per
bar

Coffee creamer (sugar-free, liquid, flavored), 0–2g net carbs
per tablespoon

Coffee creamer (sugar-free, non-dairy, powdered, flavored),
0g net carbs per teaspoon

Gum (sugar-free), 0g net carbs per stick

Hard candy (sugar-free), varies by brand, estimated 0–1g
net carbs per 4–6 pieces

MCT oil,[45] 0g net carbs per tablespoon

---

42. Hunt's 100% Natural Tomato Sauce, Hunt's Pasta Sauce (No Added Sugar), Rao's Homemade.

43. Avoid sweet and sour pickles (unless sugar-free variety).

44. Popular brands of frozen chocolate treats include Breyers CarbSmart, Enlightened, and Popsicle.

45. Not a recommended item—provided here only as a reference.

Nori, seaweed snack (roasted, salted), 0g net carbs per
5-gram serving

Popsicles (sugar-free), varies by brand, estimated 7g net
carbs per serving

Pork rinds, 0g net carbs per ½ ounce

Protein bar (Quest), 4g net carbs per bar

Tortilla[46] (low-carb), 4–6g net carbs per medium-sized tortilla

FAQS & OBSERVATIONS

After reviewing the provided grocery list, I'm sure you'll agree
there is nothing out of the ordinary here. Keto-friendly food and
drinks aren't mysterious or hard to come by. You might not have
tried these before (daikon, endive, artichoke?), but I assure you,
they are part of the norm.

- NO snobby ingredients
- NO special orders
- NO specialty (expensive) products
- NO hard-to-find items
- NO mass-produced keto-branded foods
- NO meal replacements (frozen meals, bars, shakes, pack-
aged foods)

**There is nothing extravagant here, folks! If I couldn't
find it at my local Walmart Neighborhood Market, it
didn't make it on my shopping list.**

---

46. Popular low-carb brands of tortillas include Mission Carb Balance and La Tortilla Factory Low
Carb flour tortillas.

BUT IT SAYS "KETO"

For keto beginners, I preach avoiding foods that say "keto" on the label. **I can tell you with 100% assurance that keto-labeled foods are entirely unnecessary.** More often than not, you'll find them expensive and lacking in flavor. Sure, the idea of a frozen cauliflower-crust pizza might sound promising (hold that thought for Day 6 where we discuss dirty keto foods in detail), but for now, I advise a hard pass.

COCKTAILS & CAFFEINE

Just because you want to lose weight doesn't mean you can't enjoy a cup of coffee, drink a Diet Coke, or sip a sugar-free cocktail. *Bottoms up!* You do have to be smart about it, though. The issue with drinking caffeinated[47] or alcoholic beverages lies in the aftereffects. They are all dehydrating. At the very least, they might cause you to experience mild thirst, a headache, or constipation. You might not think that's a big deal, but these symptoms often magnify once you're in ketosis.

The metabolic process of ketosis compels you to drink a sizeable amount of water to begin with (you might notice you're going to the bathroom more frequently). Expect this. What constitutes "normal," however, changes when you pile on the dehydrating effects caused by caffeine or alcohol. You've got to make amends by drinking *more*.

Yes, you can have low-carb, sugar-free caffeinated or alcoholic

---

47. Coffee, tea, sugar-free or low-carb energy drinks, diet soda.

beverages on a keto diet, but realize you must drink additional fluids and electrolytes (on top of plain water) to make up for their dehydrating effects. Compensation is the part you need to be concerned with (or endure some gnarly consequences).

🔊 **Take note: hydrate, Hydrate, HYDRATE!**

KETO FLU, I GOT YOU!

Not drinking enough water is likely to result in some discomfort. Dehydration symptoms range in complexity and severity; not everyone will experience the same symptoms. Heed the warning signs:

- Headache (mild to severe)
- Muscle cramping (especially leg cramps, often at night)
- Feelings of tiredness, exhaustion, dizziness
- Changes in urination (frequency, color, possible development of kidney stones)
- Bouts of confusion or disorientation
- The appearance of pale skin, sunken eyes or cheeks
- Dry mouth or thirst (which ironically occurs during late-stage dehydration)
- Heatstroke
- Loss of consciousness, coma, death

Collectively, the symptoms of dehydration are referred to by many as the "keto flu." It's not a badge of honor or rite of passage; it's something you *can* and *should* avoid. There's no need to suffer or put yourself at risk. I can't say this enough—*take measures to prevent this from happening.*

To reiterate, ketosis, the way your body now provides you with energy, operates using a lot of water, likely more than you're used to drinking. Balance drinking water with the right mix of electrolytes (sodium, potassium, calcium, magnesium). How this is done is not complicated.

Include sugar-free sports drinks[48] or electrolyte-enhanced waters[49] in your shopping cart. Sprinkle NoSalt[50] on your food. If you prefer a more natural approach, sip pickle juice or drink bone broth. Eat foods rich in potassium (nuts, salmon, avocado, leafy greens, mushrooms) and high in calcium (yogurt, cheese, leafy greens, broccoli, fish, almonds, coconut milk, salmon, shrimp, peanuts) while drinking plenty of water.

FAST-FORWARD TO FRUIT

Many of us mistakenly assume that fruit and weight loss go hand in hand—grapefruit diet, anyone? We've got to let go of the myth that all fruit is good for you. True, fruit is natural, but grown in soil doesn't always mean nourishing.[51] Most fruit contains high amounts of *fructose*, a type of sugar. As we've discussed, high amounts of sugar (in any form) can lead to disastrous consequences. For this reason, I suggest you enjoy lower-carb fruits in moderation (within your daily allocation of carbs). The choice is yours. See for yourself how fruits stack up.

---

48. Gatorade Zero, Powerade Zero Sugar, Propel Zero Sugar Electrolyte Beverage.

49. MiO, Propel, Smartwater.

50. NoSalt Sodium-Free Salt Alternative.

51. Opium, tobacco, mold . . . all are natural, but definitely not recommended!

KETO-FRIENDLY FRUIT COMPARISON

Fruit (sorted low to high by net carbs)	Net Carbs	Serving Size
Rhubarb	3g	1 cup
Avocado	3g	1 medium fruit
Lemon	4g	1 medium fruit
Lime	5g	1 medium fruit
Tomato	5g	1 medium fruit
Jicama*	5g	1 cup
Blackberries	6g	1 cup
Raspberries	7g	1 cup
Strawberries	8g	1 cup
Watermelon	11g	1 cup
Cantaloupe	11g	1 cup
Nectarine	12g	1 cup
Coconut (unsweetened)	12g	1 cup
Peach	13g	1 cup
Pear	15g	1 cup
Plum	16g	1 cup
Orange	17g	1 cup
Blueberries	18g	1 cup
Pineapple	19g	1 cup
Tangerine	22g	1 cup
Mango	22g	1 cup
Apple	23g	1 medium fruit
Banana	26g	1 medium fruit
Grapes	26g	1 cup

*Though technically a vegetable, because jicama tastes sweet, I'm going to take some creative license here and also include it with the list of fruits.

FRUIT FAIRNESS

You CAN eat fruit and stay in ketosis. It's all about moderation. Using a few tricks, you'll learn how to enjoy fruit without feeling punished by the restraint. Here are some of the sneaky strategies I found helpful:

Get schooled: Understanding fruit's effect on blood sugar levels puts decision-making into perspective. No one is saying that fruit is "bad." Fructose, the natural sweetener in fruit, causes a spike in glucose same as table sugar (sucrose).

Stop hatin': If having a particular fruit is imperative to your success, figure out a way to enjoy it (and avoid feeling resentment).

Little bit: With fruit, moderation is what matters. Reduce the serving size by serving as a topping instead of an individual snack (like berries on yogurt). Or, pre-portion amounts of fruit in food storage containers.

Pump the brakes: Frozen fruit alone, or added to your drink in ice cubes, makes a creative, chilled treat that can't be rushed!

Fruity faux flavoring: Please a passion for fruit flavors with an artificial substitute (i.e., sugar-free gum, flavored protein powder, or water flavor enhancer).

Color explosion: Add small amounts of fruit to a smoothie for flavor and color. If needed, add additional sugar-free flavored gelatin powder for a boost.

Fresh to death: Compared to frozen or canned fruit (which is often drenched in sugary syrup anyway), fresh fruit offers the most bang for your buck in terms of flavor.

Tick-tock: Timing is everything. Eat fruit before planned exercise to allow your body an opportunity to metabolize it (as opposed to before sleep).

LOW-CARB FRUIT

CHEAT-SHEET FOR FRUIT
HOW MANY NET CARBS IN ONE CUP?

Rhubarb
3g

Avocado (pureed)
5g

Starfruit
5g

Tomato (chopped)
5g

Jicama
5g

Blackberries
6g

Raspberries
7g

Strawberries (whole)
8g

VEGETABLE VULNERABILITY

Just like fruit, not all vegetables can be treated equally. Would you guess that a large baked potato and a 2-pack of chocolate Hostess cupcakes both have 50 grams of carbs? (*Soooooooooooo* not fair, I know.) Starchy vegetables like corn, potatoes, peas, and carrots contain surprisingly higher carbs than lettuce, broccoli, or asparagus. The numbers speak for themselves. It's not pretty! Study the provided chart to see what I mean.

KETO-FRIENDLY VEGETABLE COMPARISON

Vegetables (sorted high to low by net carbs)	Net Carbs	Serving Size
Cassava	60g	1 cup
Plantains	54g	1 cup
Potatoes (white)	50g	1 cup
Yams	33g	1 cup
Corn	25g	1 cup
Water chestnuts	25g	1 cup
Potatoes (sweet)	23g	1 cup
Parsnips	21g	1 cup
Pumpkin (mashed)	16g	1 cup
Peas (green)	13g	1 cup
Onions (red, yellow, white)	12g	1 cup
Rutabaga	12g	1 cup
Bell pepper (red)	12g	1 cup
Artichokes	10g	1 cup
Beets	9g	1 cup
Bell pepper (yellow)	8g	1 cup
Turnips	8g	1 cup
Carrots	8g	1 cup
Squash (spaghetti)	8g	1 cup
Squash (winter, acorn, butternut, pumpkin)	8g	1 cup
Okra (cooked from fresh)	7g	1 cup

KETO-FRIENDLY VEGETABLE COMPARISON

Vegetables (sorted high to low by net carbs)	Net Carbs	Serving Size
Brussels sprouts (cooked from fresh)	6g	1 cup
Jicama	5g	1 cup
Bell pepper (green)	4g	1 cup
Broccoli (fresh)	4g	1 cup
Green beans (string)	4g	1 cup
Squash (summer, zucchini, yellow, green)	3g	1 cup
Tomatoes*	5g	1 medium fruit
Cabbage (green)	3g	1 cup
Cauliflower	3g	1 cup
Asparagus	2g	1 cup
Cucumbers	2g	1 cup
Eggplant	2g	1 cup
Mushrooms	2g	1 cup
Celery	1g	1 cup
Lettuce	1g	1 cup
Zucchini	1g	1 cup
Spinach	0g	1 cup
Alfalfa sprouts	0g	1 cup

*Though technically a fruit, tomatoes are frequently used as a vegetable in cooking.

Start by eating the low-carb vegetables you like (even if there's only one!) and go from there. You don't have to love or eat them all.

Once you see the weight loss effects of replacing french fries with low-carb veggies, you might become increasingly motivated to try more of them. Have an open mind. You might shock yourself.

 Observing the scale move in a favorable direction has an extraordinary way of reducing vegetable anxiety.

FULL-FAT FABULOUSNESS

No low-fat or fat-free products exist in ANY of my recipes or grocery lists. Those unsatisfying foods are a thing of the past. *Good riddance.* How long has it been since you enjoyed legit butter? Dipped an artichoke leaf in real mayonnaise? For some, never. (The judgment, the shame!) Wake up those taste buds. Savor traditional cuts of meat, avocados, nuts, cholesterol-filled eggs, and full-fat dairy products. Finally, REAL food.

Fat makes everything better. It puts a smile on your face. You're much more likely to continue with a way of eating when the food is fantastic *and* fills you up.

With DIRTY, LAZY, KETO, there is no macro goal to reach each day for eating fat (none for protein, either). This means *you don't need to eat fat for fat's sake to hit a targeted number* (a stereotypical mistake among beginners and strict keto dropouts). When it comes to fat, use common sense. Going overboard with fat bombs (and the like) often results in a weight loss stall or gain. **Remind yourself constantly:** *a fat fixation will not spur ketosis!*

 Don't be afraid of fat, but use it strategically. Fat can transform healthier food (like vegetables) from dreary to divine.

HIGH-FAT, LOW-CARB FOODS

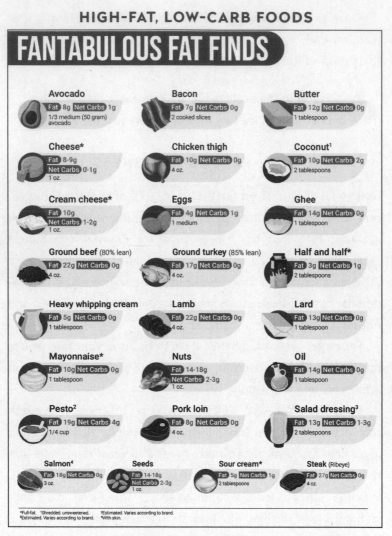

FANTABULOUS FAT FINDS

Avocado
Fat 8g Net Carbs 1g
1/3 medium (50 gram) avocado

Bacon
Fat 7g Net Carbs 0g
2 cooked slices

Butter
Fat 12g Net Carbs 0g
1 tablespoon

Cheese*
Fat 8-9g
Net Carbs 0-1g
1 oz.

Chicken thigh
Fat 10g Net Carbs 0g
4 oz.

Coconut[1]
Fat 10g Net Carbs 2g
2 tablespoons

Cream cheese*
Fat 10g
Net Carbs 1-2g
1 oz.

Eggs
Fat 4g Net Carbs 1g
1 medium

Ghee
Fat 14g Net Carbs 0g
1 tablespoon

Ground beef (80% lean)
Fat 22g Net Carbs 0g
4 oz.

Ground turkey (85% lean)
Fat 17g Net Carbs 0g
4 oz.

Half and half*
Fat 3g Net Carbs 1g
2 tablespoons

Heavy whipping cream
Fat 5g Net Carbs 0g
1 tablespoon

Lamb
Fat 22g Net Carbs 0g
4 oz.

Lard
Fat 13g Net Carbs 0g
1 tablespoon

Mayonnaise*
Fat 10g Net Carbs 0g
1 tablespoon

Nuts
Fat 14-18g
Net Carbs 2-3g
1 oz.

Oil
Fat 14g Net Carbs 0g
1 tablespoon

Pesto[2]
Fat 19g Net Carbs 4g
1/4 cup

Pork loin
Fat 8g Net Carbs 0g
4 oz.

Salad dressing[3]
Fat 13g Net Carbs 1-3g
2 tablespoons

Salmon[4]
Fat 18g Net Carbs 0g
3 oz.

Seeds
Fat 14-18g
Net Carbs 2-3g
1 oz.

Sour cream*
Fat 5g Net Carbs 1g
2 tablespoons

Steak (Ribeye)
Fat 27g Net Carbs 0g
4 oz.

*Full-fat.   [1]Shredded, unsweetened.   [3]Estimated. Varies according to brand.
[2]Estimated. Varies according to brand.   [4]With skin.

PROTEIN POWER

Like fat, protein takes longer for the body to break down and digest. Besides protecting muscle mass, it also helps you to feel full. *This is wonderful!* Use this phenomenon to your advantage. I bet you'll find that you do less snacking after finishing a protein-rich meal.

With DIRTY, LAZY, KETO, the protein strategy isn't complicated. On the contrary, it's extra easy. *Include a hefty serving of high-protein, low-carb food at every meal, and you'll be good to go.* Here are ten ideas to get you started.

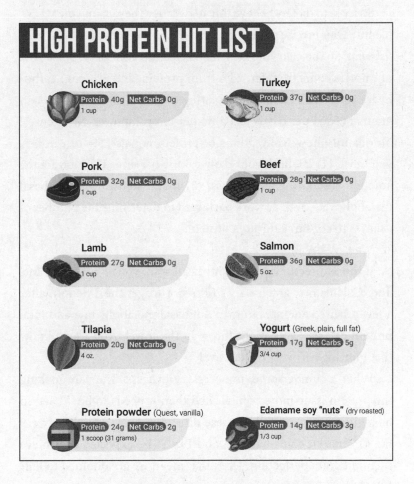

HIGH PROTEIN HIT LIST

Chicken
Protein 40g   Net Carbs 0g
1 cup

Turkey
Protein 37g   Net Carbs 0g
1 cup

Pork
Protein 32g   Net Carbs 0g
1 cup

Beef
Protein 28g   Net Carbs 0g
1 cup

Lamb
Protein 27g   Net Carbs 0g
1 cup

Salmon
Protein 36g   Net Carbs 0g
5 oz.

Tilapia
Protein 20g   Net Carbs 0g
4 oz.

Yogurt (Greek, plain, full fat)
Protein 17g   Net Carbs 5g
3/4 cup

Protein powder (Quest, vanilla)
Protein 24g   Net Carbs 2g
1 scoop (31 grams)

Edamame soy "nuts" (dry roasted)
Protein 14g   Net Carbs 3g
1/3 cup

PROTEIN PUSHBACK

Does my recommended protein strategy sound too good to be true? It's simple; I'll give you that. Straightforward explanations are often the most effective. I understand you might be hesitant to do an about-face on what you've been previously taught. Further, you might have concerns about getting too little or too much protein in your diet. *Could there be such a thing as a "perfect" amount?*

Strict keto dieters believe this to be true. They claim you MUST identify your precise protein goal and then make it happen—*no matter what.* So sharpen your pencil and clear off your desk. Since 70% of calories come from fat, 25% from protein, and 5% from carbohydrates on the keto diet, calculating the exact amount of protein grams needed per day is just a matter of brainpower. No excuses! To quantify how many grams of protein equals 25% of calories, you must: (1) establish your daily caloric baseline, (2) subtract the amount needed for weight loss, (3) make adjustments for basal metabolic rate, and (4) work backward to determine the number of calories to consume through protein.

Wait. WHAT?

If those directions made your head spin, you're not alone. Me. Too. Calculators, graph paper (let's not forget the Tylenol), after a few misfired attempts to map out basal metabolic rate and total protein calories, you might throw in the towel. And we all know that quitting isn't very productive!

What a cumbersome, unnecessary process. They are making the protein issue more complicated than it needs to be. I tried to be a guinea pig and follow these directions, but I didn't get very far. Ordinary people like you and I can't be expected to achieve such nutrition perfection. Does that mean we are doomed to fail? I don't think so!

There's no need to do a bunch of drawn-out math equations to calculate needed protein. DIRTY, LAZY, KETO makes this process intuitive.

Just like spending more money on groceries doesn't buy your way to weight loss, doing advanced keto calculus won't guarantee results. There's a much simpler way to get into ketosis (and eat the amount of protein your body needs). Follow the *Extra Easy Keto* system (no math—woo hoo!), where common sense plays a starring role. See for yourself how streamlined it is.

To start, include high-protein, low-carb food at every meal. Pay attention to hunger cues and make adjustments as needed. DIRTY, LAZY, KETO keeps the protein component extra easy—no busy-work macronutrient monitoring involved.

HIGH-PROTEIN, LOW-CARB FOODS

Meat (sorted high to low by protein)	Protein	Net Carbs	Serving Size
Pork	20–25g	0g	4 oz.
Chicken	19–25g	0g	4 oz.
Beef	19–23g	0g	4 oz.
Turkey	19–21g	0g	4 oz.
Lamb	19g	0g	4 oz.
Sausage, pork (link/patty)	14g	0–1g	3 oz.
Chicken (canned, white meat)	13g	0g	3 oz.
Lunch meat	9g	0–2g	2 oz.
Seafood	**Protein**	**Net Carbs**	**Serving Size**
Salmon (cooked from fresh)	36g	0g	5 oz.
Tilapia (cooked from fresh)	20g	0g	4 oz.
Cod (cooked from fresh)	17g	0g	4 oz.
Sardines (canned)	14g	0g	3 oz.

Seafood	Protein	Net Carbs	Serving Size
Shrimp (cooked from fresh)	12g	2g	3 oz.
Tuna (canned in oil)	11g	0g	2 oz.

Nuts	Protein	Net Carbs	Serving Size
Edamame soy "nuts" (dry roasted)	14g	3g	⅓ cup
Peanuts (shelled)	7g	3g	¼ cup
Almonds	6g	3g	¼ cup
Pistachios (roasted with shell)	6g	5g	½ cup

Seeds	Protein	Net Carbs	Serving Size
Hemp seed hearts (shelled hemp seeds)	10g	0g	3 tablespoons
Pumpkin (pepitas) (unshelled)	8g	2g	¼ cup
Sunflower (unshelled)	6g	4g	¼ cup
Flaxseed (whole)	6g	2g	3 tablespoons
Sesame (raw, hulled)	5g	4g	¼ cup
Chia (black, whole)	4g	0g	2 tablespoons

Dairy	Protein	Net Carbs	Serving Size
Yogurt (Greek, plain, full-fat)	14g	5g	¾ cup
Cottage cheese, 4% milkfat	12g	5g	½ cup
Soy milk (unsweetened)	8g	2g	1 cup
Cheddar cheese (full-fat, block)	7g	0g	1 oz.
Mozzarella (whole milk, shredded)	7g	1g	¼ cup
Eggs	6g	0–1g	1 egg

Soy	Protein	Net Carbs	Serving Size
Edamame soy "nuts" (dry roasted)	14g	3g	⅓ cup
Textured vegetable protein	12g	5g	¼ cup
Black soybeans (Eden brand)	11g	5g	½ cup
Soybeans (edamame, shelled)	11g	3g	½ cup
Soy milk (unsweetened)	8g	2g	1 cup
Tofu	6g	0g	3 oz.

Miscellaneous	Protein	Net Carbs	Serving Size
Protein shake (Premier brand)	30g	2–3g	1 shake (11.5 fl. oz.)
Protein powder (Quest brand, vanilla)	24g	2g	1 scoop (31 grams)
Protein bar (Quest brand)	20g	4g	1 bar
Chicken (canned, white meat)	13g	0g	3 oz.
Jerky (beef)	11g	6g	1 oz.
Lunch meat	9g	0–2g	2 oz.
Peanut butter	7g	6g	2 tablespoons
Pepperoni	5g	0g	15 slices (28 grams)
Salami	5g	0g	1 oz.
Hot dog (beef)	4g	0–1g	1 link (42 grams)

PROTEIN PERFECTION

Forcing yourself to meet a daily protein goal (even if you're not hungry or doing just fine with weight loss) makes no sense. Why overcomplicate something so instinctual? Plus, obsessively following orders won't teach you to listen to your body's cues. How completely illogical!

Unless you're consuming a lot of protein powder or meal replacement bars, protein doesn't usually lend itself to overeating. It's probably the *least* tempting of the three macronutrients.[52] (Rarely is the person seduced into eating plate *after plate* of grilled chicken.) It's more likely that you don't eat enough protein or don't eat it often enough. If your weight loss has stalled, or you find yourself feeling hungry between meals, pay attention to *how much* protein you're eating and *when*. (Up the amount and or frequency.) A little more protein, or perhaps more often throughout the day, might be all the nudge you need.

Is there a minimum amount of protein you need to eat? For what it's worth, the recommended daily allowance (RDA) of protein intake for adults is roughly 10 to 35% of total caloric intake.[53] Multiply your weight (in pounds) by 0.36 to figure out what this means for you. Here's the equation for a 150-pound woman: 150 x 0.36 = 54 grams of protein. Does that seem like a lot? Don't let this "requirement" intimidate you. Heed my advice about eating *some* protein at every meal, and this minimum threshold can easily be met (no graph paper required).

PROTEIN PROOF

Take a look at the provided chart of high-protein, low-carb foods. Circle a choice for breakfast, lunch, dinner, and a snack. I'll

---

52. As a reminder, the three macronutrients are fat, protein, and carbohydrates.

53. Paula Trumbo et al., "Dietary Reference Intakes for Energy, Carbohydrate, Fiber, Fat, Fatty Acids, Cholesterol, Protein and Amino Acids," *Journal of the Academy of Nutrition and Dietetics* (November 2002).

give you a sample, continuing with the hypothetical 150-pound woman. As you can see, eating a minimum amount of protein (in this case, 54 grams) is not something we need to chart or stress out over. It adds up rather quickly.

Breakfast: egg (6 grams), sausage (14 grams)
Lunch: lunch meat (9 grams)
Dinner: beef patty (19 grams)
Snack: almonds (6 grams)
Total protein = 54 grams

CUSTOM KETO

From protein to produce, remember this: *you* are in control of what is on your plate. That said, don't fret if you have a favorite food or drink that hasn't been discussed yet. The provided lists of foods here are not all-encompassing. You are allowed to add more. A little due diligence is all that's called for when deciding what makes the cut on DIRTY, LAZY, KETO.

A review of the product's Nutrition Facts label will ease your conscience and help you make an educated decision about eating any given food. My de facto rule of thumb has always been "10 or less" (under 10 grams net carbs per serving). *Avoid temptation, I say!* There's nothing wrong with being conservative, especially when starting. After all, borderline higher-net-carb foods often lead to trouble.

Customize keto on your terms. Whether you're dealing with a specific food allergy, think you hate a particular vegetable, or self-identify as a picky eater, recognize that everyone has some challenge or another about food. No one will force you to eat an avocado (or any other food you don't like). If you're allergic to eggs or nuts, don't eat them. It's as simple as that. Design the lifestyle to work *for you.*

Getting past your unique situation might take extra effort. Hang tight. You might have to get creative. With hard work and determination, anything is possible. Don't let selective eating or food allergies, for example, hold you back (or become an excuse). Achieving your goals is totally worth it!

CORNER STORE KETO

We're almost halfway through the week. It's exciting to see it all come together. You learned which foods support ketosis, and are now equipped to take the next step. *Field trip!* This errand won't take long. DIRTY, LAZY, KETO foods are within reach no matter where you live. A traditional grocery store is your one-stop shop.

Feel empowered as you decide what to put in your shopping cart. There are plenty of options available. No matter your preferences or limitations, know you can tailor this way of eating and make it your own. You're making excellent progress. Eat, drink, shop—repeat!

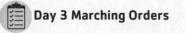 **Day 3 Marching Orders**

1. *Build a balanced list of favorites from the provided starter grocery lists. Add any desired appropriate items not listed.*
2. *Think about how your personal preferences or food chal-*

lenges might impact shopping or cooking on DIRTY, LAZY, KETO. How will you adjust?

3. *Describe your plan to stay hydrated. Be sure to address alcohol and caffeine.*

4. *Smile! Grocery shop with an open mind and positive attitude.*

DAY 4: MEAL PLANNING

Today you'll unlock the ketogenic meal-planning mystery. *Ooooh! Ahhhh!* (It's exciting, I know!) I'll teach you my secret system: a convenient and clever strategy for balancing macronutrient distribution that entails very little work on your part (unless you count doing dishes). Building mouth-watering, keto-friendly meals will soon become second nature. *No scary keto math is required.*

What's the first step to making meal planning easier? Focus on the proven keto basics—then STOP. Avoid complicated recipes for now. There are plenty of low-maintenance breakfast, lunch, and dinner options available. Choose recipes with limited ingredients while you gain confidence. **Conventional meals, quick-fix snacks . . . keto doesn't have to be elaborate to work.** *And that's a win!*

Stop overthinking the keto weight loss formula. You don't need a spreadsheet or calculator to make dinner. Sit back and relax. There's no need to micromanage the number of calories or exact macronutrients on your plate. Expect details like these to be built into the DIRTY, LAZY, KETO process.

GOOF-PROOF PLAN

Meals that support ketosis draw from the **Big Three**—healthy fats, lean protein, and slow-burning vegetable carbs. So simple! Embrace the *Extra Easy Keto* meal-planning strategy and avoid mathematical rigamarole. There's no need to stress about meeting exact macronutrient ratios (that's strict keto nonsense); an imperfect method also gets the job done. Meals conceived with the Big Three are tasty and filling. In a word: yummy! Fat, protein, and slow-burning, non-starchy vegetables digest *slowly* in the gut. The overall experience is pleasurable.

THE BIG THREE

FAT	PROTEIN	VEGETABLE CARBS
avocado, butter, cheese, cream, olives, oil	steak, chicken, egg, shrimp, tofu, bacon	asparagus, broccoli, cauliflower, cucumber, lettuce, mushrooms

KETO COLLABORATION

The proof is in the pudding. Eating meals constructed with the Big Three components leads to weight loss. Hunger pains? Diminished. There's less snacking between meals. You won't feel deprived, either. Higher-fat meals are rich and indulgent. Behind the scenes, the combination of higher fat, steady protein, and lower-carb foods maintains a state of ketosis. Your metabolism burns body fat as its fuel. Each of these points, individually and in tandem, makes regulating body weight possible (our little metabolic miracle). *Hip, hip, hooray!*

The Big Three work as a team to help you lose weight. Balance is key. Too much of one player, or not enough of the other, is likely to run afoul (read—weight loss stall or gain). Mind your keto Ps and Qs to prevent this from happening.

KETO CONDUCT

Eating too much fat at once: Fats, especially "fat bombs,"[54] can be overly enticing. It's hard to stop! Overeating fat in one sitting (without protein and veggies to balance out the meal) can cause immediate stomach upset, diarrhea, and, ultimately, weight gain.

Eating fat "just because": Ignore this bad advice circulating on social media. You don't need to eat spoonful after spoonful of fat to lose weight on a keto diet. That doesn't make sense! Eating fat— for no reason at all—is likely to cause weight *gain*, not loss.

> ⚠ Ketosis (fat-burning mode) is brought on by restricting the availability of carbs in your system (*not* by eating fat).

Skimping on fat: The fat-free, low-fat diets from the 1980s are as passé as leg warmers. Even the Mayo Clinic agrees that including fats in our diet gives us energy and helps us digest essential vitamins.[55] Omitting fats from your meals won't do you any favors. Fat is needed to keep you satiated (both emotionally and physically) throughout the day.

> 📢 Fat isn't the solo artist here. The Big Three band is a trio. Combine fat, protein, and vegetable carbs to make your metabolism sing.

---

54. Keto slang for a high-fat, sugar-free dessert.
55. www.mayoclinic.org/healthy-lifestyle/nutrition-and-healthy-eating/in-depth/fat/art-20045550.

Responding to hunger cues (or lack thereof): The effect of the Big Three on your metabolism is emotionally and physically gratifying. Most people report not feeling hungry in between meals. Not snacking is new! Without conscious effort, serving sizes get smaller. This pleasant revelation catches some people off guard. *They worry something is wrong with them!* Eating less food, less often, is to be expected. It's a positive sign. Your body is learning how to crave *only* the nourishment it actually needs.

Can't stop eating: If you're challenged with overeating (due to habit, not hunger), make a conscious effort to fill up with foods that are high in fiber (low-carb veggies, fruits, nuts, and seeds). Fiber is a type of complex carbohydrate that takes a while for your body to digest (which keeps you from roaming the kitchen). You'll end up eating less food, less often.

> **Gradually increase the amount of fiber in your diet to avoid gassiness and stomach upset.**

Avoiding all *vegetables*: Strategically use fats in your diet to make "healthier" food (like vegetables) more appealing. Slap some butter on just about anything, and *BAM!*—you'll want more. Foods prepared with fat taste rich, decadent even. You certainly won't "feel" like you're on a diet (for many of us, this matters).

Not eating enough *fiber*: Fiber is the gift that keeps on giving. High-fiber carbs serve as a low-impact filler for a hard-to-fill tummy. Don't pass up this opportunity! Fiber physically helps stop you from overeating (or becoming preoccupied) with other, riskier foods. There is simply no room for more. It improves overall digestive health (and prevents constipation). *You can thank me later.*

Agonizing over vegetable carbs: Here's the truth. Not one of us became overweight from vegetables. They aren't the villain here—so eat up, friends. Because of their high fiber content, non-starchy, slow-burning vegetables expand in the gut. They physically slow you down from eating more food (critical for those of us who lack an off switch). I can't think of a better way to spend your carbs!

📢 **EEK!** *Soooooo many vegetables?* **Don't let yourself get overwhelmed. Hone in on the word "ideally" (and take baby steps).**

Overloading protein: Some people expressed concerns that overeating protein leads to weight gain. True, a surplus of protein will metabolize into glucose, but to be blunt, for most of us, that doesn't explain a sudden increase on the scale. A more likely effect of too much protein is constipation. Listen to what your body is telling you. Irregularity is a sign that you need to make a change. Reduce protein intake, drink more water, walk, and increase slow-burning vegetable carbs.

Fearing protein: Undereating protein has its share of problems too. You'll likely feel hungry in between meals. A severe lack of protein can lead to hair loss or damaged nails.[56] The consequences of eating "too much" protein far outweigh the cost of not eating enough. At the minimum, include a serving of high-protein, low-carb food at every meal.

Focusing on protein goals: You don't need to obsess about counting grams of protein or meeting precise macronutrient goals

---

56. Hair loss does not always indicate a protein deficiency. It may be related to a hormone imbalance (like hypothyroidism) or something more temporary, like the body reacting to a sudden diet change. Always consult with your health care provider to address any medical concerns.

(that's strict keto busywork). The DIRTY, LAZY, KETO strategy is more instinctual. What does your body need? When eaten regularly, high-protein, low-carb foods curb hunger. Include some at every meal and be done with it. That's it? *Yep.* Task, complete.

> ⚠ **Eat when you're hungry. Stop eating when you're full. You don't need to "get your fats in" or force yourself to reach an arbitrary protein goal. We're trying this in a new way. Practice learning to listen to your body's needs.**

COMPLETE KETO KIT

Have you had any "aha" moments about the Big Three strategy? It's so exciting when that inner light bulb turns on and you see the full picture. I GET IT! If you're not quite there yet, try visualizing what this looks like on a plate. See how fat, protein, and vegetable carb foods come together in these popular low-carb meals.

- Grilled steak with a side of buttered broccoli
- Cobb salad with ranch dressing
- Vegetable-stuffed omelet topped with bacon bits
- Fajita chicken strips with sliced bell pepper and guacamole
- Hamburger patty topped with sauteed mushrooms
- Pesto shrimp and zucchini noodles
- Lettuce-wrapped deli meat and cheese "un-wich" with a dill pickle
- Porkchop and mashed cauliflower with low-carb gravy
- Grilled salmon with a side of green beans sprinkled with almond slivers

- Vegetarian stir-fry—tofu and chopped asparagus sauteed in oil
- Egg scramble with spinach, tomato, and feta cheese
- Protein smoothie (spinach, berries, protein powder, unsweetened dairy-alternative milk)
- Tuna fish salad (canned tuna, mayo) with celery sticks
- Your turn! Name three ideas.

EASY-PEASY PLANNING

Did you notice the above meals contain very few ingredients? The modesty was intentional. *We're in the learning phase here, people.* Everyone can benefit from a quick refresher of the keto basics. Go through the above list and practice categorizing foods as fats, protein, or vegetable carbs. A grilled steak would be a *protein*, while a side of buttered broccoli is a *vegetable carb* topped with *fat*. Feel free to flip back to earlier resources for help. Soon, mixing and matching foods for meal-building will become as foolproof as getting dressed in Garanimals.[57]

One of my favorite dinners consists of a supermarket rotisserie chicken served with salad (from a bag) and ranch dressing. Dinner's ready *(in under a minute)*. BAM!

Way to go! You've mastered the Big Three basics. (That wasn't so hard, was it?) Go on to the next level and flex your knowledge. Discover how it all fits together by tackling a full day's menu.

---

57. A popular US brand of children's clothing that started in the 1970s, the Garanimals line helped children get dressed "all by themselves" with mix-and-match separates (themed animal tops and bottoms).

MENU MEAL CHALLENGE

Sample menus A, B, and C describe typical days on DIRTY, LAZY, KETO. Take a moment and study each meal and snack. Task yourself with picking out the Big Three foods. Choose which category *best* describes each ingredient: FAT, PROTEIN, or VEGETABLE CARB. Next, estimate (or look up) net carbs per ingredient (single standard serving size, unless indicated otherwise). Add up the total number of net carbs per meal/snack/day. Lastly, note any questions or concerns that come up along the way. Verify your answers after each section. Keep practicing until you get the hang of it. *Piece of cake!*

Sample Menu A

Breakfast: (_____ g net carbs): Two scrambled eggs fried in butter served with a side of bacon. Coffee (with heavy whipping cream and sugar substitute) and water to drink.

Snack: (_____ g net carbs): Cucumber rounds dipped in ranch dressing. Sugar-free lemonade to drink.

Lunch: (_____ g net carbs): Lettuce-wrapped "un-wich" with deli meat, cheddar cheese, and mayonnaise. Served with a dill pickle. Diet soda and water to drink.

Snack: (_____ g net carbs): Handful of pecans.

Dinner: (_____ g net carbs): Roasted turkey breast and mashed cauliflower with gravy, served with a side of buttered green beans. Herbal iced tea (unsweetened) to drink.

Dessert: (_____ g net carbs): Sugar-free flavored gelatin with a squirt of whipped dairy topping from a can.

Total (estimated): _____ grams of net carbs

ANSWERS: SAMPLE MENU A

Breakfast: (3g net carbs): Two scrambled eggs (PROTEIN) fried in butter (FAT) served with a side of bacon (PROTEIN). Coffee (with heavy whipping cream [FAT] and sugar substitute) and water to drink.

Eggs, 1g net carb per egg

Butter, 0g net carbs per tablespoon

Bacon, 0g net carbs per 2 slices

Coffee (black), 0g net carbs per 8 fl. ounces

Heavy whipping cream, 0g net carbs per tablespoon

Sugar substitute (monk fruit, sucralose, Stevia, etc.), 0g net carbs per packet

Water (flat), 0g net carbs per 8 fl. ounces

Snack: (4g net carbs): Cucumber rounds (VEGETABLE CARB) dipped in ranch dressing (FAT). Sugar-free lemonade to drink.

Cucumber, 2g net carbs per cup

Salad dressing (ranch), 1g net carb per 2 tablespoons

Lemonade-flavored drink enhancer, sugar-free, 1g net carb per ½ packet

Water (flat), 0g net carb per 8 fl. ounces

Lunch: (2g net carbs): Lettuce-wrapped (VEGETABLE CARB) "un-wich" with deli meat (PROTEIN), cheddar cheese (FAT), and mayonnaise (FAT). Served with a dill pickle (VEGETABLE CARB), diet soda, and water.

Lettuce leaves (romaine), 0g net carbs per 3 leaves

Deli meat (varies by brand), estimated 1g net carbs per 2 ounces

Cheddar cheese, 1g net carb per ounce

Mayonnaise (full-fat), 0g net carbs per tablespoon

Diet soda, 0g net carbs per 8 fl. ounces

Water (flat), 0g net carbs per 8 fl. ounces

Snack: (1g net carb): Handful of pecans (FAT).

Pecans (halves), 1g net carb per ¼ cup

Dinner: (9g net carbs): Roasted turkey breast (PROTEIN) and mashed cauliflower (VEGETABLE CARB) with gravy (FAT), served with a side of buttered green beans (VEGETABLE CARB, FAT). Herbal iced tea (unsweetened) to drink.

Turkey, 0g net carb per 3 ounces

Cauliflower (riced), 2g net carbs per ½ cup

Gravy (turkey), 3g net carbs per ¼ cup

Green beans (string), 4g net carbs per cup

Butter, 0g net carbs per tablespoon

Iced tea (unsweetened, sugar-free, herbal), 0g net carbs per 8 fl. ounces

Dessert: (1g net carb): Sugar-free flavored gelatin with a squirt of whipped dairy topping from a can.

Gelatin, prepared (sugar-free, any flavor), 0g net carbs per ½ cup

Whipped dairy topping in a can (regular), 1g net carb per
  2 tablespoons

Total (estimated): 20 grams of net carbs

Sample Menu B

Breakfast: (_____ g net carbs): Yogurt (flavored with vanilla
and sugar-free sweetener) topped with macadamia nuts. Coffee
and water to drink.

Snack: (_____ g net carbs): Zucchini slices coated with grated
Parmesan cheese with a sugar-free sports drink.

Lunch: (_____ g net carbs): Tuna salad (canned tuna, mayonnaise) eaten with celery stalks. Sparkling water with lime to drink.

Snack: (_____ g net carbs): "Anti-pasta" bowl with pepperoni,
olives, cherry tomatoes, salami, and mozzarella cheese cubes. Water
to drink.

Dinner: (_____ g net carbs): Beef and broccoli stir-fry over
cauliflower rice. Red wine and mineral water to drink.

Dessert: (_____ g net carbs): A few squares of 85 to 86% chocolate.

Total (estimated): _____ grams of net carbs

ANSWERS: SAMPLE MENU B

Breakfast: (7g net carbs): Yogurt (PROTEIN/FAT) (flavored with
vanilla and sugar-free sweetener) topped with macadamia nuts
(FAT). Coffee and water to drink.

Yogurt (5% milkfat, Greek, strained, plain), 5g net carbs per
  ¾ cup

Vanilla (pure), 0g net carbs per ⅛ teaspoon

Sugar substitute (monk fruit, sucralose, Stevia, etc.), 0g net
carbs per packet

Macadamia nuts, 2g net carbs per ounce

Coffee (black), 0g net carbs per 8 fl. ounces

Water (flat), 0g net carbs per 8 fl. ounces

Snack: (2g net carbs): Zucchini slices (VEGETABLE CARB)
coated with grated Parmesan cheese with a sugar-free sports drink.

Zucchini (raw), 1g net carb per cup

Parmesan cheese, 1g net carb per ounce

Sugar-free sports drink,[58] 0g net carbs per 8 fl. ounces

Lunch: (1g net carb): Tuna salad—canned tuna (PROTEIN), mayonnaise (FAT)—with celery stalks (VEGETABLE CARB). Sparkling water with lime to drink.

Tuna (canned in oil), 0g net carbs per ¼ cup

Mayonnaise (full-fat), 0g net carbs per tablespoon

Celery (raw), 1g net carb per cup

Water (sparkling), 0g net carbs per 8 fl. ounces

Lime juice, 0g net carbs per teaspoon

Snack: (5g net carbs): "Anti-pasta" bowl with pepperoni (PRO-
TEIN), olives (FAT), tomatoes (VEGETABLE CARB), salami
(PROTEIN), and mozzarella cheese cubes (FAT). Water to drink.

---

58. MiO, Gatorade Zero, Powerade Zero Sugar, Smartwater.

Pepperoni, 0g net carbs per 15 slices

Olives (black), 1g net carb per 2 large olives

Tomato (cherry), 2g net carbs per 3 cherry tomatoes

Salami, 1g net carb per 5 slices

Mozzarella cheese cubes, 1g net carb per ounce

Water (flat), 0g net carbs per 8 fl. ounces

Dinner: (9g net carbs): Beef (PROTEIN) and broccoli (VEGETA-BLE CARB) stir-fry over cauliflower rice (VEGETABLE CARB). Red wine and mineral water to drink.

Beef, 0g net carbs per 3 ounces

Broccoli (fresh), 4g net carbs per cup

Oil, 0g net carbs per tablespoon

Cauliflower (riced), 2g net carbs per ½ cup

Red wine (pinot noir), 3g net carbs per 5 fl. ounces

Mineral water or naturally flavored water (sugar-free), 0g net carbs per 8 fl. ounces

Dessert: (6g net carbs): A few squares of 85 to 86% chocolate.

Cacao, 85 to 86% chocolate, 6g net carbs per 2½ pieces (30 grams)

Total (estimated): 30 grams of net carbs

Sample Menu C

Breakfast: (_____ g net carbs): Cottage cheese topped with blueberries. Coffee and water to drink.

Snack: (_____ g net carbs): Celery stalks dipped in peanut butter. Diet soda and water to drink.

Lunch: (_____ g net carbs): Traditional Cobb salad (lettuce, chicken, egg, avocado, blue cheese, cherry tomatoes, bacon, dressing). Water to drink.

Snack: (_____ g net carbs): Steamed artichoke leaves dipped in mayonnaise. Water to drink.

Dinner: (_____ g net carbs): Grilled salmon with roasted Brussels sprouts cooked in oil. Beer (low-carb) and water to drink.

Dessert: (_____ g net carbs): Trail mix (almonds, sugar-free chocolate chips, unsweetened shredded coconut).

Total (estimated): _____ grams of net carbs

ANSWERS SAMPLE MENU C

Breakfast: (14g net carbs): Cottage cheese (PROTEIN) topped with blueberries. Coffee and water to drink.

Cottage cheese, 4% milkfat, 5g net carbs per ½ cup
Blueberries, 9g net carbs per ½ cup
Coffee (black), 0g net carbs per 8 fl. ounces
Heavy whipping cream, 0g net carbs per tablespoon
Sugar substitute (monk fruit, sucralose, Stevia, etc.), 0g net carbs per packet
Water (flat), 0g net carbs per 8 fl. ounces

Snack: (7g net carbs): Celery stalks (VEGETABLE CARB) dipped in peanut butter (FAT). Diet soda and water to drink.

Celery (raw), 1g net carb per cup

Peanut butter, 6g net carbs per 2 tablespoons

Diet soda, 0g net carbs per 8 fl. ounces

Water (flat), 0g net carbs per 8 fl. ounces

Lunch: (9g net carbs): Traditional Cobb salad—lettuce (VEGETA-BLE CARB), chicken (PROTEIN), egg (PROTEIN), avocado (FAT), blue cheese (FAT), double serving of cherry tomatoes (VEGETA-BLE CARB), bacon (PROTEIN), dressing (FAT). Water to drink.

Salad greens (lettuce mix), 1g net carb per 2 cups

Chicken, 0g net carbs per 3 ounces

Egg (hard-boiled), 1g net carb per egg

Avocado, 1g net carb per ⅓ of a medium avocado

Blue cheese (crumbles), 1g net carb per ¼ cup

Cherry tomatoes, 4g net carbs per 6 cherry tomatoes

Bacon (unflavored), 0g net carbs per 2 cooked slices

Salad dressing (blue cheese), 1g net carb per 2 tablespoons

Water (flat), 0g net carbs per 8 fl. ounces

Snack: (5g net carbs): Steamed artichoke leaves (VEGETABLE CARB) dipped in mayonnaise (FAT). Water to drink.

Artichoke, 5g net carbs per ½ cup

Mayonnaise (full-fat), 0g net carbs per tablespoon

Water (flat), 0g net carbs per 8 fl. ounces

Dinner: (9g net carbs): Grilled salmon (PROTEIN) with roasted Brussels sprouts (VEGETABLE CARB) cooked in oil (FAT). Beer (low-carb) and water to drink.

Salmon, 0g net carbs per 3-ounce fillet

Brussels sprouts (cooked from fresh), 6g net carbs per cup

Oil, 0g net carbs per tablespoon

Beer (low-carb), 3g net carbs per 12 fl. ounces

Water (flat), 0g net carbs per 8 fl. ounces

Dessert: (6g net carbs): Trail mix—almonds (FAT), sugar-free chocolate chips, unsweetened shredded coconut (FAT).

Almonds, 3g net carbs per ounce

Chocolate chips (sugar-free, sweetened with monk fruit[59]),
    1g net carb per 60 chips (14 grams)

Coconut (unsweetened, shredded), 2g net carbs per 2 tablespoons

Total (estimated): 50 grams of net carbs

CARB-COUNTING CLARITY

Take a time-out and check for understanding. Think about how you did with each menu challenge. Are you proficient now in calculating net carbs? Could you correctly identify the Big Three in meals? The goal here wasn't perfection—it was practice. Optimistically, the repetition helped! Perhaps you uncovered an area that needs more review. Or maybe your level of accuracy was surprising? Either way, I expect this task was worth your time. At the very least, you now have three days of meals and snacks ready to go.

---

59. ChocZero, Lakanto, Lily's Sweets.

I have to ask. During the activity, did you find yourself thinking, *The quantity! There's* A LOT *to eat here* (which can be a shocker for some). *You don't need to starve yourself to lose weight.* Further, you probably noticed how each sample menu contained inconsistent amounts of total net carbs (A = 20, B = 30, C = 50). The spread was intentional. As we've discussed, there are a variety of circumstances that influence how many net carbs each person can eat in ketosis.

I wanted you to see just how comfortable meal planning can be. Shop where you feel comfortable and buy low-carb foods you genuinely like. There is such a wide variety of flavorful foods at your fingertips. Prioritize personal preferences to make DIRTY, LAZY, KETO meal planning achievable and compelling; otherwise, why bother?

The next step is putting your plan into action. The only thing stopping you is, well, *you!*

KETO SMARTER (NOT HARDER)

Setting your standards too high regarding meal prep or expecting your "bad" habits to change overnight is likely to backfire. Not knowing what to eat for breakfast is a prime example. For many, indecision can cause dietary paralysis. *Might as well pour a bowl of Frosted Flakes.* Talk about unproductive!

Setting unreachable expectations for yourself regarding home cooking (frequency, limiting choices to purely organic, cooking wholly from scratch) is a recipe for disappointment, maybe even failure. Think about Know-it-all Keto Karen. She couldn't keep up! Idealism comes at a cost. Maybe in a perfect world, all our meals would be homemade (with preservative-free, farm-raised, locally sourced ingredients), but that *ain't gonna happen* for most of us.

And that's okay.

> ⚠️ **Spending MORE money on groceries won't help you lose MORE weight any faster.**

Your pocketbook and on-the-go schedule don't have to be at odds with achieving weight loss goals. Flexibility and cost matter when deciding what to eat. Wouldn't you agree? Do your best while being realistic. Don't beat yourself up for hitting up the drive-thru or reaching for a gourmet coffee (if that's your thing). Both actions can be done under the guise of healthy eating. There is no right or wrong way to execute a DIRTY, LAZY, KETO meal plan. Do what is comfortable for you (and get out of your own way).

LOW-CARB LICKETY-SPLIT

Don't be shy about cutting corners for meal prep; include convenience food in your grocery shopping (but be sure to read the Nutrition Facts labels). You don't have to make every meal from scratch. Stop being so hard on yourself. Embrace more down-to-earth standards and watch DIRTY, LAZY, KETO become effortless. Here are some examples:

- bagged lettuce or spinach
- pre-washed, pre-cut fresh vegetables
- rotisserie chicken, plain—no barbeque sauce
- flash-frozen meats (individually portioned)

- deli meat
- frozen riced cauliflower
- shredded coleslaw
- canned pasta sauce (no sugar added)
- peeled hard-boiled eggs
- shredded or sliced cheese
- canned meat (tuna, chicken, Spam, etc.)
- packaged to-go salads
- pre-minced garlic
- precooked meats (sausage, bacon)
- frozen berries
- precooked, peeled, and cleaned frozen shrimp
- starter sauces (alfredo, pesto, no-sugar-added marinara)
- frozen zoodles (zucchini noodles)
- drive-thru burgers (bunless, of course)
- canned or frozen vegetables
- individually portioned/packaged foods (string cheese, nuts, etc.)

📢 **Learn how to work with your eating or cooking habits (not against!) and you'll be shopping for smaller clothes.**

FLAWED & FABULOUS

Aside from stressing about how often to cook and what ingredients to use, many people become stuck trying to fix their other "bad" eating habits. They waste time and energy trying to become a different person. Which of these descriptions applies to you?

I rarely eat breakfast (but I know I'm supposed to).
Oh, my sweet tooth!
Late-night snacker? Yep, that's me.
Where's the kitchen? I hardly ever cook.
No time to cook—I'm always on the go.
I need a pick-me-up! (I get so sleepy.)
I'm such a BIG eater.
I snack all the time (even when not hungry).
For my schedule, eating one big meal a day makes sense.
I'm so picky. I HATE vegetables (or eggs, avocados, etc.).
I can't live without X (Pepsi, rice, tortillas, etc.).
I mostly eat out.

Everyone has quirks about food. There is nothing wrong with you liking sweets or enjoying a snack in front of the TV. *Just be you!* Stop spinning your wheels by trying to reverse decades of so-called "problematic" behaviors, and instead, *MODIFY*. Learn to go with the flow.

When you let go of "*shoulds*" and the "*shouldn'ts*," you'll finally stop *sh^*+ing* on yourself—ha!

You don't need to feel ashamed about your eating habits. Adding regret to the stir of other emotions you're likely experiencing is counterproductive. As I shared in the opening, my DIRTY, LAZY, KETO journey included learning to accept all parts of myself (even if that meant eating dessert for breakfast). I mean *really*. Who cares?

REALISTIC WORKAROUNDS

Name your so-called "bad" eating habits or preferences. If not mentioned here, by all means, add them to the list. Don't spend too much time on this activity (the negativity can suck you in!). Identify areas of concern, then *chop-chop*. Force yourself to move on. Spend your energy devising a creative workaround.

Below, I've matched up classic habits and preferences with keto-friendly solutions. Do any appeal to you? If not, think of viable alternatives. Chances are, there's a way to work with your current behaviors while staying on the plan. Be specific. Part of your Day 4 marching orders includes making a modification plan. How will you sidestep any potential snags?

Habit/Preference	Solution
Likes to skip breakfast	Practice intermittent fasting (IF)
Craves a sweet after dinner	Plan for a sugar-free dessert
Tends to eat a late-night snack	Set aside some carb spend for the evening
Lacks interest in home cooking	Prioritize shortcut meals when grocery shopping
Always pressed for time	Set up low-carb grab-and-go snacks/meals
Needs a quick boost	Enjoy a low-carb or sugar-free caffeinated drink
Returns for seconds (and thirds!)	Prepare low-carb dishes that yield larger portions
Happier eating one meal a day (OMAD)	Be strategic with macronutrients

Frequently munches on a snack	Keep low-carb/zero-carb foods close by
Maintains *this* food is a must-have	Find a copycat recipe or low-carb equivalent
Mostly dines out	Choose restaurants and order meals on plan

> ⚠️ **Don't try to outrun your sweet tooth. It's likely to catch up and give you a "snack"-down.** *Bahahaha!*

KETO PROGRESS, NOT PERFECTION

Your journey is bound to have setbacks. Expect hiccups. *You're human!* When mistakes happen, forgive yourself (then dive back in). Resist sexy shortcuts (egg fasts, meal replacement bars or shakes, ketone drinks). You can do this on your own.

Focus on the basics. Putting together a homecooked meal that supports weight loss doesn't have to be complicated. Think *Extra Easy Keto*. Rely on the Big Three to carry the burden for you and make meal planning more manageable.

 Conquer one meal at a time. Today, roasted chicken, tomorrow—the world!

Have patience with yourself while you learn a new way of eating. Be kind. Stay positive. Embrace idiosyncrasies instead of trying to "fix" them. Developing new skills (and gaining keto-confidence) takes time and practice. Your efforts will be rewarded. The gifts of DIRTY, LAZY, KETO last a lifetime!

Day 4 Marching Orders

1. *Explain the function of the Big Three. Name at least six meals that illustrate this concept.*
2. *Complete the Menu Meal Challenge. Practice calculating net carbs for accuracy.*
3. *Pinpoint your top five "troublesome" eating habits. Put into place a workaround plan for each.*

DAY 5: ROUTINES

Have you ever been out to eat with one of those health nuts who *NEVER* seems to struggle over what to order? They superficially look over the menu—for a few seconds, mind you—and predictably fall head over heels for a plain (humdrum), heart-smart entree. (They don't even scan the dessert menu. *What-ava!*)

"I'll have the [plain-Jane, no fun] X," they order with conviction.

Why couldn't I be more like that?

Meanwhile, I sit there wavering, feeling terrible about my wants versus needs. I'll hold up the whole table while I deliberate about what to order.

Should I, or shouldn't I?

When I first started "dieting," temptation followed me everywhere. I *literally* sat on my hands in restaurant booths (hoping physical restraint would prevent me from getting into trouble). My mind would start racing.

Pancakes or eggs . . . PANCAKES or eggs . . . A GOLDEN STACK OF WARM, FLUFFY, BUTTERY PANCAKES WITH MAPLE SYRUP or, *sigh* . . . eggs?

I did a lot of hemming and hawing back in those days. Like a fool, I put all of my faith in willpower alone. Boy, was that stressful! I couldn't trust myself to do the "right" thing. I expected that making responsible decisions would be *effortless*. (Where did I get *THAT* idea?)

Still, I crossed my fingers, hoping circumstances would eventually change. Maybe with enough time, dieting wouldn't be so hard. If the stars aligned just so, would motivation and willpower finally fall into place?

"*UNLIKELY!*" said my Magic 8 Ball.

KETO COOL UNDER PRESSURE

There had to be a better way. If I couldn't depend on my instincts for proper guidance, I'd have to look elsewhere. Surely, the answer existed. Hard and fast rules about nutrition didn't work for me, that I knew. Nonetheless, I needed some semblance of order. Instead of obsessing over every morsel of food, I'd focus all my energy on developing better overall habits.

Ignore the palate. Stick to the plan.

Fake it 'til ya make it.

(Can you believe THIS was my big idea?)

It's pathetic what prompted me to go in this direction because it started more than twenty years ago (apparently, I'm a slow learner).

I was observing a kindergarten class as part of my student teaching. In spite of not being able to read and being so young, the children were able to perform a number of complicated tasks, often flawlessly. From correctly putting away art supplies to swiftly finding assigned spots on the rug, their little five-year-old brains were programmed to follow expectations. They knew where to go and when without a single chaotic moment. The class was practically on autopilot.

The lack of stragglers or complainers fascinated me. How was this possible? From cleanup to lineup, the children automatically marched along. The teacher didn't bark orders; she didn't say a word. They practiced these drills from the very beginning. Rituals, not rules, built order from chaos.

That's what I needed to do.

ROUTINES ROCK (RULES NOT!)

Routines, not dieting rules, would help me eliminate the guesswork about what to eat. Should I or shouldn't I? There would be no decision-making at all! No drama, less trauma. If I wanted to build long-lasting habits, *THIS* was the answer. A premeditated plan.

Rules	Routines
Apply the same to everyone	Can be tailored for the individual
Rigid	Flexible
Boring	Allow for creativity
"All or nothing" mentality	Adaptable
Can cause rebellion	Encourage choice
Can be intimidating	Provide reassurance (encourage confidence)
Following correctly can be traumatic	Comforting during times of stress

KETO QUICKSAND

You might be hesitant about having too much structure. Will having so many protocols in place feel constricting? At least for me, this hasn't been the case. Compared to punitive dieting rules, I've found rituals comforting. They bring me feelings of relief. I don't stress as much about slipping up. **Having a plan helps avoid heat-of-the-moment decision-making.** In turn, I get less worked up about food choices. I can finally relax and get the job done.

Nobody wants to lose weight only to gain it back again. Stop relying on motivation or willpower alone (it has a tendency to fizzle out). Forgo this insanity and try a fresh perspective.

You know that I lost 140 pounds, but keep in mind, that's only half of my story. DIRTY, LAZY, KETO also helps me maintain that weight loss (going on a decade!). None of this happened by accident. Routines helped me target my problem areas. For me, this meant not having enough time, money, or focus. My excuses sounded something like this.

I don't have enough time to (cook, grocery shop, meal-prep, pack a lunch, or exercise).
I can't afford those ingredients.
I'm too (tired, stressed, or overwhelmed) to deal with this now.
I don't know how.
Maybe later.
I have too much going on (at work, with the family).
I don't wanna.

Reflect on your past. What type of roadblocks do you put up that stop you from eating healthier? Make a list of the excuses you tell yourself (but don't stop there). Look for any underlying themes. Then try and connect the dots. What routines could address your issues? Yes, this is only the first week of DIRTY, LAZY, KETO, but we're playing the long game here. This is your destiny. *Take charge!*

CAPTAIN KETO

Extra Easy Keto routines are your savior for long-term success. Day 5 includes concrete examples with how-to (often entertaining) advice. You might snicker—*is she for real?* I assure you that these habits are legit. (I'll show you my costume closet.) I try to make tasks playful whenever feasible. From grocery shopping to meal prep and cleanup, DIRTY, LAZY, KETO doesn't have to be *borrrrrrrrring*.

These hacks took time to develop. Lucky you, this is a step you can skip. No sense in having to figure out this stuff on your own. Steal my ideas shamelessly. Tweak them as you see fit. Get inspired and kick off protocols of your own. Do whatever you have to do to get yourself into a low-carb groove. Ready to rock and roll? Let's start at the top.

> **Routines are like lifeguards for choosing what to eat. They can prevent you from drowning—*don't get in the water without them!***

1. I don't have enough time.

Enjoy theme nights: Take the guesswork out of tonight's dreaded kitchen duty. "What's for dinner?" isn't a burden when you include theme nights in your meal planning. With Taco Tuesday, Fried Chicken Friday, or Soup Sunday on the docket, half the week's meals are basically done. (Winning!) No one even notices you had the same thing last week when there is a spirited twist on the menu (especially when you wear a silly outfit or play theme music). It's hysterical too. (My kids might disagree, but whatever, I'm the one cooking!)

Cook fast: Speed up cooking whenever possible. Make mouth-watering meals using kitchen appliances like the air fryer (cook meat from frozen!)—then tidy up in a flash. Reduce time spent prepping by incorporating nifty time-saving ingredients sold at the grocery store (microwavable packaging, pre-washed vegetables, starter sauces, and more).

QUICKIE KETO COOKING TOOLS

- air fryer (try using a disposable liner—*genius!*)
- pressure cooker (Instant Pot)
- microwave
- waffle maker (chaffle maker)
- wok
- convection oven
- broiler
- gas grill
- oven bag
- double broiler
- deep fryer

Spend up: Invest in your kitchen (and your health). Spend money on convenience foods or time-saving cooking gadgets that will help you become more efficient.

Set it in stone: Vow to meal-prep tasks on a locked-in timetable. Plan on doing the same "chores" on the same day and time each week. Then you'll never have to fret about finding the time or a willing participant. Lock it into your to-do list and *get 'er done* on autopilot (grocery shopping, prepping vegetables for the week, enjoying a night off, etc.).

🔊 **Failing to plan is a plan to fail.**

Shop the edge: Shorten your grocery store trips by following this rule: shop the store's perimeter. Almost everything you need is along the building's four walls (stores usually stock perishables here). Avoid wandering up and down the aisles to save time and ward off temptation.

All together now: Prepare meals in less time by cooking needed ingredients simultaneously. Tools like the slow cooker, pressure cooker, or even sheet pans will do the heavy lifting for you. You won't have to juggle multiple pots and pans. Cleanup becomes a breeze when there is one pot to wash (or stuff in the dishwasher).

Press replay: When you find a meal or snack that works, have it again. And again. Enjoy the same thing for breakfast every day if that is your preference (Martha Stewart is not watching). Make favorite recipes often. Stop trying to reinvent the wheel and relax.

Shop online: Stop driving in circles and shop for groceries online. The time you'll save! Take advantage of free delivery or curbside pickup. You have better things to do than deal with traffic or wait in long lines (like packing a lunch for tomorrow or whipping up tonight's dinner).

Get automated: Duplicate purchase? Save yourself the trip. Set up a standing order with autopay and autoship (how lazy is

THIS!). At my house, bulk orders of lemon-flavored sugar-free gelatin (among other random ingredients) are automatically delivered every ninety days (yes, I eat that much Jell-O).

Cancel Betty Crocker: Embrace meal-making shortcuts as the new norm. Off-the-shelf convenience foods are valuable time-savers (and worth every bit of added expense if they help you stay committed). Don't judge yourself harshly. Who says you must make every component of a meal from scratch? Sorry, mom. "Homemade" means "made at home," in my opinion (in any shape or form).

STORE-BOUGHT KETO TIME-SAVERS

- lettuce mix (pre-washed)
- coleslaw mix (pre-washed)
- broth (canned, carton)
- spinach (pre-washed)
- cheese (shredded, sliced, sticks)
- cauliflower (riced, frozen)
- rotisserie chicken
- bacon (precooked crumbles, strips)
- single portions of meat (individually wrapped, flash-frozen)
- pasta sauce, no sugar added (canned)
- bell pepper medley fajita mix (frozen)
- spice blends (ranch, Greek, taco seasoning, steak seasoning)
- hard-boiled eggs (peeled)
- sausage (precooked)[60]

---

60. Aidells.

- kebabs (premade)
- berries (frozen strawberries, blueberries, etc.)
- assorted fresh vegetables (pre-washed/cut, ready-to-eat, microwavable packaging)
- assorted canned vegetables (green beans, mushrooms, asparagus, etc.)
- assorted frozen vegetables (broccoli, Brussels sprouts, cauliflower, etc.)
- spinach dip
- pesto
- alfredo sauce

Dinner for one: Individually portioned meats, like flash-frozen chicken breasts or salmon fillets, make cooking for one person more efficient. On the rare occasion when I cook myself something different from the rest of the family (not because the keto diet requires a special meal, only when I don't like what they're having), I pop a single serving of meat in the air fryer (frozen, no less!).

> ⚠️ **Start with minor changes, then see them through. Aim for consistency when following DIRTY, LAZY, KETO routines, not perfection. It's the seemingly inconsequential decisions that end up mattering the most. *Mark my words.***

Be an early bird: Decide on meals a day (or more) in advance. Planning gives you more time to gather the ingredients you need (with the fringe benefit of making you *feel* focused and productive). I've gotten into the habit of deciding the next day's dinner before bed. I pull out the prescribed ingredients from the pantry and start thawing meat in the fridge. Sometimes, I'll wake up in the morning, see everything laid out, and feel motivated to start cooking dinner earlier in the day (which I'll later reheat).

Don't be fresh: Don't be snobby about ingredients (leave that for the strict keto people). Produce doesn't always have to be expensive, organic, or fresh to be nutritious. What's available (at the store and in your kitchen) counts too. Be flexible. Include frozen or canned ingredients to save yourself time, money, and unnecessary driving around town. You can't beat the convenience of shopping "at home." Less waste too.

CANNED KETO PRODUCE
- artichoke hearts
- asparagus
- chiles
- green beans
- hearts of palm
- jalapeños
- olives
- pumpkin
- mushrooms
- spinach
- tomatoes

FROZEN KETO PRODUCE
- avocado chunks
- blueberries
- broccoli florets
- Brussels sprouts

- cauliflower (riced, florets)
- edamame
- green beans
- collard greens
- raspberries
- spinach
- strawberries
- zucchini "noodles"

One and done: Prep ingredients for the week en masse (as opposed to before every meal). Clean and cut multiple days' worth of fresh vegetables in one sitting—then grab on the run later. Cook larger portion sizes of meat (to enjoy over multiple meals). Label and freeze the remaining ingredients for use in upcoming recipes.

Now and later: Cook extras of your favorites to enjoy again later. It's like a BOGO. Whenever I bake egg bites, I increase the recipe and freeze extra portions. Toss in the microwave and VOILA! Breakfast, served. Lazy or efficient? Who cares. I always find meals more enjoyable when no prep work is involved.

2. I can't afford it.

Love your leftovers: Don't turn your nose up. Reinventing leftovers will save you oodles of time, money, and sanity. Keep a Rolodex of possibilities on hand (keep photos on your phone) and use them often.

Stack it, pack it, and rack it: It's not enough to say, *I'll store this food for later*. Refrigerated food tends to get lost in the back-of-the-fridge abyss (or maybe that only happens at my house?). Aim to become more organized. Stackable, see-through food storage containers will help you locate items instantaneously. There's less spoilage too. You'll be more inclined to eat leftovers in a timely fashion when the packaging looks more attractive.

Double down: Why make one DIRTY, LAZY, KETO dinner when you can easily make two? Freeze the second dish to enjoy later (your future self thanks you). Apart from being a time-saver, making meals in bulk is more economical. Another idea is to partner up with a like-minded friend—who's also on the low-carb bandwagon—and trade duplicate meals. (Be sure to text me her number!)

Can it: Including canned products makes sense—lots of cents (sorry, I couldn't help myself). Look beyond the typical can of green beans. Incorporate canned meats, fish, starter sauces, and convenience foods in your meal planning.

CANNED MISCELLANEOUS KETO FAVORITES
- broth
- chicken
- clams
- crab (not imitation)
- coconut milk (unsweetened, 12 to 14% fat)
- enchilada sauce (red, green)
- olives
- pasta sauce (no sugar added)[61]
- salsa
- sardines
- sausage

---

61. Hunt's 100% Natural Tomato Sauce, Hunt's Pasta Sauce (No Added Sugar), Rao's Homemade.

- soybeans (black)[62]
- spam
- tuna

Shop sales: Stretch your grocery budget by taking advantage of discounted prices. Plan meals around seasonal and on-sale ingredients. Don't be afraid to stock up your pantry or freezer. Frequently used items won't go to waste. I'm not scared of using six-month-old frozen shredded mozzarella—*are you?*

Buy it frozen: Take advantage of cost-saving opportunities like buying in bulk, catching a discount sale, or storing leftovers. If necessary, buy a second freezer (and a thick pair of mittens for when you need to dig to the bottom). With food safety in mind (plus a little organization), you'll be able to extend the shelf life of all your necessities.

FREEZER FINDS

Open my freezer on any given day and here's what you'll see:
- bacon
- cheese (shredded)
- desserts (individually portioned, low-carb)
- fish (salmon, shrimp)
- ice (crushed) for making smoothies
- ice cream (low-carb)
- leftovers
- meats (individual flash-frozen items and in larger units)
- popsicles (sugar-free)
- produce (low-carb vegetables and berries)

---

62. Eden.

Buy in bulk: You don't need a big family or a small business to warrant warehouse grocery shopping. Not every item sells in a mega-sized volume. Even with standard grocery items, discounts here can be steep. Warehouse shopping can help you save cash when you know what to buy.

CLUB KETO (WAREHOUSE)[63]

- alcohol (spirits)
- almond flour (super-fine, blanched)
- bacon
- cheese, hard (shredded, sliced)
- cheese, soft (cream cheese, feta, goat)
- chicken (rotisserie)
- deli-style lunch meat
- eggs
- heavy whipping cream
- oil
- pickles
- produce, fresh (artichokes, avocados, broccoli, lettuce)
- produce, frozen (berries, riced cauliflower)
- nuts (raw)
- nut butter (peanut butter, almond butter)
- protein shakes (low-carb)
- meat and seafood
- sauce
- sports drinks (sugar-free, electrolyte-enhanced water)
- unsweetened, dairy alternative milk (low-carb)
- water (bottled)

---

63. Costco, Walmart Supercenter, Sam's Club.

Do it yourself: Saving both time *and* money regarding food prep can be a toss-up. Often, it's either one or the other. Take a brick of cheese. Shredded or sliced cheese will probably cost more at the register when compared to the price of a brick. Now I realize that some of you might fear the potato starch in mass-produced shredded cheese (added to prevent caking). Still. Do you have the time or energy to shred or slice cheese by hand? If so, more power to you. You'll be able to pocket a few bucks (while getting a free workout). Either way, know that a smidge of potato starch won't break the bank or your keto goals.

Shop around: If following a tight budget, make time to comparison shop. Visit multiple stores. Take advantage of loss leaders and price matching at each store. Register for store emails and loyalty programs and study their offerings. Plan meals around what foods are in season or on sale. Ask for a raincheck when discounted items temporarily go out of stock. Don't be shy about asking for help. (Hint: stalk employees that carry a mark-down gun.) Where there is a will, there is a way!

Include restaurant food: Eating on the go doesn't have to be stressful. You're even allowed to eat fast food on DIRTY, LAZY, KETO (don't let the strict keto bullies tell you otherwise). Relish the many new options. It's all about pre-planning. Make informed choices by educating yourself about a restaurant's menu.[64] Take your time and speak up for yourself when ordering. Be assertive about what you want to be added or subtracted from your meal. You're paying for it!

Here's what self-advocacy can sound like:

---

64. Need help finding nutritional information about restaurant food? Check out the *Keto Diet Restaurant Guide* (2022) or *DIRTY, LAZY, KETO Fast Food Guide: 10 Carbs or Less* (2018), both by William and Stephanie Laska.

I'll have double the protein on my salad—yes, that's fine to charge me extra.

Please wrap my burger with lettuce leaves (no bun, thanks).

No beans or rice in my chicken bowl. I'll have extra veggies added instead.

I'd like my coffee drink made with heavy whipping cream, please (not milk).

Who's in charge of what you eat? You are!

3. I'm too overwhelmed (stressed) right now.

Schedule it: Avoid feeling angst about a looming task by setting aside time in the future to get it done. This isn't procrastination. You're taking action (and it feels less scary). This strategy helped me when I first started exercising. I was terrified! Scheduling my "start" was a productive first (baby) step.

Tackle priorities first thing in the morning. Obvious? Not to me! I couldn't bear to admit it was true. Exercise, drinking water, prepping vegetables . . . *at sunrise?* (I don't exactly wake up thinking about celery.) Still. I've learned to do these things right away before the excuses take over.

Kitchen is closed: Speaking of scheduling, one of the more constructive routines I ever crafted was shutting down my kitchen for the night, starting immediately after dinner. At least at my house, I finally realized there was nothing decent about my late-night snacking (it only spelled T-R-O-U-B-L-E). Call it intermittent fasting if you'd like; I say the kitchen is closed.

Check yourself (or wreck yourself): How do you spend your time these days? In the wake of COVID, I found myself backsliding. The amount of television binge-watching I was doing? Let's just say there was a permanent dent on my couch. I know my stress levels decrease automatically by spending time outdoors (not mindlessly snacking in front of the television). I didn't shame myself for slipping. Instead, I went for a walk. Immediately, I felt better! When things get out of whack, don't hesitate to make a swift change.

📢 For me, waiting until the end of the day to try and exercise is pointless. *Not gonna happen* (my excuses are real doozies!). I've learned to put on my exercise clothes first thing in the morning—no matter what.

Protect & prioritize: Revere the time you devote to self-care (meal prep, grocery shopping, exercise) just as you would a doctor's appointment. I've learned to treat them with equal importance. No canceling allowed. Watch out for tempting competing offers (which are just veiled excuses). Remind yourself what's most important—taking care of YOU.

On the go: I won't even go to the mailbox without food or drink in hand. Why? Because leaving the sanctity of your kitchen can feel like you're entering the Wild West. Who knows what food "dangers" might be lurking on your trail or how long you'll be gone? Brace yourself for a DIRTY, LAZY, KETO snack attack. Pack a lunch pail or insulated cooler for the ride. Here are some "travel-friendly" ideas.

KETO TO GO

Cheese stick, 1g net carb per stick (28 grams)

Jerky, dried meat (varies by brand), estimated 5–6g net carbs per ounce

Zucchini spears, 1g net carb per cup

Celery stalks, 1g net carb per cup

Yogurt cup (5% milkfat, Greek, strained, plain), 5g net carbs per ¾ cup

Cucumber rounds, 2g net carbs per cup

Hard-boiled egg, 1g net carb per egg

Cauliflower florets (raw), 3g net carbs per cup

Deli meat (varies by brand), estimated 1g net carbs per 2 ounces

Canned meat (Spam, Vienna sausage, etc.), 1–2g net carbs per 2 ounces

Pickles (dill), 1–2g net carbs per ¾ spear (1 ounce)

Protein bar, low-carb (Quest brand), 4g net carbs per bar (200 grams)

Bell pepper (green), sliced, 4g net carbs per cup

Pepperoni, 0g net carbs per 15 slices (28 grams)

Olives (black), 1g net carb per 2 large olives

Nut butter or peanut butter (no sugar added), 3–6g net carbs per 2 tablespoons

Nori, seaweed snack (roasted, salted), 0g net carbs per 5-gram serving

Strawberries, 8g net carbs per cup

Cheese crisps, 1g net carbs per ounce

Sunflower seeds (unshelled), 3g net carbs per ¼ cup

Pork rinds, 0g net carbs per ½ ounce

Blueberries, 5g net carbs per ¼ cup

Nuts (macadamia, peanuts, almonds, walnuts, pecans), 1–3g net carbs per ounce

Hard candy (sugar-free), varies by brand, estimated 0–1g net carbs per 4–6 pieces

Gum (sugar-free), 0g net carbs per stick

Edamame (shelled), 3g net carbs per ½ cup

Fast food side salad, 2g net carbs per small side salad[65]

Tortilla (low-carb), 4–6g net carbs per medium-sized tortilla

Bottled water, 0g net carbs per 8 fl. ounces

Water with flavored drink enhancer, sugar-free, 0–3g net carbs per serving[66]

Diet soda, 0g net carbs per 8 fl. ounces

Energy drink (sugar-free or low-carb), 0–3g net carbs per 8 fl. ounces

Coffee (black), 0g net carbs per 8 fl. ounces

Tea (unsweetened, sugar-free: herbal, black, green), 0g net carbs per 8 fl. ounces

Protein shake (low-carb, ready to drink), 2–3g net carbs per 11½ fl. ounces

Sports drink (sugar-free, electrolyte-enhanced water), 0–1g net carbs per 8 fl. ounces

Emergency stash: I probably stress about food more than most, but in the event of an emergency, I feel comfort in having a backup plan. No matter where you are—home, work, car—store low-carb nonperishables to help you weather the storm (literally!).

---

65. https://fastfoodnutrition.org/mcdonalds/side-salad

66. Serving sizes vary among brands.

> ⚠️ Just like an asthmatic has a backup rescue inhaler, I keep low-carb essentials on hand for emergencies. I realize being *hangry* isn't a life-threatening condition, though it feels like a 911 situation to me. I don't want to dwell on food all the time. Knowing I have a hidden stash keeps me from feeling anxious.

Breezy recipes: When I'm tired, the last thing I want to do is cook a complicated meal. I've learned to select basic recipes—the fewer ingredients, the better. By removing any barriers (lengthy directions, exotic or expensive ingredients, etc.), I'm much more likely to follow through.

> ⚠️ Don't let "perfect" be the enemy of "good enough." Pinterest food-prep images (Ball jar salads, Bento boxes filled with nuts and cheese) can be intimidating!

Limit frequency: Set achievable expectations about how often you're willing to meal prep. You don't have to cook every day. There's nothing wrong with going out to eat (just make low-carb choices). I usually cook two or three big meals a week, filling in the gaps by eating leftovers.

Eat out: Reduce your stress levels by regularly taking a night off from home cooking (notice I didn't say a night off from DIRTY, LAZY, KETO). Learning *how to eat out* is equally as valuable as learning *how to cook*: research the restaurant's menu[67] before you go. Decide what to order ahead of time.

---

67. For ideas of what to order, look inside the *Keto Diet Restaurant Guide: Eat Healthy & Stay in Ketosis, Dining Out on a Low Carb Diet* by William and Stephanie Laska (2022).

⚠️ **Avoid keto burnout from trying to do too much, too often. Take a night *off* from the kitchen—enjoy a *keto-licious* meal out on the town!**

RESTAURANT KETO CUISINE

Keep these go-to low-carb entrees in your hip pocket for your next meal out.

American: Bunless burger; steak with vegetables

Chinese: Grilled fish with vegetables (no sauce)

Greek: Greek salad (no pita); gyro (no bun)

Indian: Butter chicken; chicken tikka masala; tandoori chicken (no rice or naan)

Italian: Antipasti; minestrone (no noodles); fish with vegetables

Japanese: Edamame; miso soup; sashimi (no rice)

Mexican: Fajitas (no rice, beans, or tortillas); guacamole (no chips); shrimp cocktail (*coctel de camarones*)

Thai: Curry with steamed vegetables (no rice)

Vietnamese: Pho (no noodles)

One for all: There is no need to make yourself (or anyone else) a special meal. *Who has time for that?* Higher-fat, low-carb foods are enjoyable, after all. There is nothing weird or "diety" going on here. I mostly serve dishes family style. Like at a buffet, each person chooses what food to put on their plate.

If a family member demands potatoes for dinner (or rice, pasta, etc.), teach them how to boil water. *For heaven's sake!* They can learn how to make it themselves. Stop enabling others.

Prevent last-minute errands: Maintain par levels of indispensable, routine ingredients. What foods can you NOT live without? (I gotta have my cucumbers and feta!) Keep a grocery list of what's needed to make upcoming meals. Utilize technology to help with reminders. Take a picture of tonight's recipe or ask Alexa to put something in your shopping cart.

Right in front of you: Keep ready-to-eat snacks within reach and at eye level. Reorganize your fridge, pantry, and even your desk, and remove (even the most minor) obstacles. Remove or tuck away higher-carb foods. (I stash them in tall cabinets I can't reach.) Your goal is to make the healthiest choice more attractive.

Dump the gunk! Toss irresistible high-carb foods. You can't eat what's not there.

Delegate more: Free up more time for yourself with a divide-and-conquer strategy of dividing the workload among all family members (cooking, cleaning, shopping, etc.). Message to self: I'm a mom, not a maid!

ROUTINE WRAP-UP

The takeaway lesson of Day 5 is to stop depending on willpower alone to help you lose weight. She's a fickle friend, there for you *when she feels like it*. Managing your weight is an around-the-clock job. You need a trustworthy source of support. Unlike self-control (which waxes and wanes), pre-planned routines will never let you down. You'll find they make a much better bestie!

> Once I got started, the payback was immediate. Solid habits replaced guesswork. I stopped wasting time. I felt energized. *Focused.* In hindsight, having a plan in place (*what to eat* and *when to eat it*) was a no-brainer. There was no stress over what to do next. My self-esteem and weight loss accelerated. The strategy became a game-changer. To my amazement, making better decisions about what to eat became second nature, even automatic.

Day 5 Marching Orders

1. *Think about challenging aspects of weight loss; what areas concern you the most? Develop personalized routines to target these areas.*
2. *Agree or disagree: Following a default plan can prevent impulsive (and regretful) decisions later. Explain your reasoning.*
3. *From the get-go, practice your* Extra Easy Keto *routines (again and again).*

DAY 6: PLAY DIRTY

Welcome to the realm of "dirty keto"—a fantasy land where you can have your (sugar-free) cake and eat it too. Artificial sweeteners and low-carb substitutes are fair game, as are grain-based fillers, chemical additives, and even alcohol (cheers!). Freedom of choice separates DIRTY, LAZY, KETO from the rest. Even better, *you* make the rules. **Dirty keto encompasses more than just unorthodox food—it describes a flexible, judgment-free approach to low-carb eating.**

Hello! Now you're talking my language.

CUT LOOSE & KETO

We haven't spent much time discussing packaged sweets or commercial "keto" contraband items until now. Early on, I hinted there would be a little wiggle room with DIRTY, LAZY, KETO. I'm going to follow through on that promise.

Low-carb ice cream, pizza, beer? Are sugar-free candies or diet soda REALLY allowed?

Absolutely. These playful foods (and more) fall within the provocative jurisdiction of dirty keto (which, for most, is an area wildly misunderstood). My opinions on the matter are controversial—cover your eyes, Keto Karen—what comes next might get risqué.

There is nothing wrong with embracing convenience or wanton desires. A little variety can spice things up! You *don't* have to go without. I believe you should include dirty keto foods in your diet in some form or another. (Best. News. Ever.)

We need to stop shunning this topic. Dirty keto foods are not categorically beneath us. What you call dirty, I call options. Be willing to mull over both sides of the issue before making up your mind. *Don't throw the baby out with the bathwater.* When used wisely, dirty keto options can be integral to your weight loss journey. There's a lot of value here. At the very least, they offer a much-needed backup plan.

Admittedly, the freedom to enjoy dirty keto foods comes with a hefty responsibility. There are pros and cons to every situation—not all of us can (or should) indulge in dirty keto foods in the same way. (I wish it were so cut and dry.) For some, low-carbs treats (ice cream, chips) are a slippery slope. On the other hand, there are a whole lot of folks unaffected by their charm. Either way, the situation is fluid. *Personal.* Striking a balance between "all or nothing" when enjoying dirty keto foods and "once in a while" can be tricky. That doesn't mean their merits aren't worth exploring.

QUESTIONABLE KETO

This topic is so high-priority that we'll spend an entire day on it, starting now. We'll explore all of your questions. Will dirty keto foods stop weight loss? What are the benefits and drawbacks?

How do you trouble-shoot temptation? Guidance is provided for when (and why) to switch gears. By the end of Day 6, you'll have a roadmap for how best to drive forward.

But I don't eat fast food . . . or junk food.

Okay, okay. I anticipated at least one holdout. There's always one person who assumes this type of food doesn't apply to them. They want permission to jump ahead, skipping over this section altogether. *That's not gonna happen.* Nevertheless, stay with me here anyway. Here's why.

You may not eat fast food. However, that's not all we're going to talk about today. Take to heart dirty keto foods again, but this time, think bigger. Let go of the media's portrayal. The dirty keto umbrella covers much more than what's being served at your local drive-thru.

THAT'S NOT KETO!

Dirty keto foods run the gambit from what you might expect— traditional junk food—all the way to produce, like pre-packaged salads. That's right, SALADS! Processed food encompasses all sorts of innocent goodies. A package of frozen cauliflower, a can of green beans? At least in my mind, if it ever hit the assembly line, it counts as *dirty*. From artificial flavors and colors to shelf-stable additives or convenient packaging, ready-to-eat dirty keto foods may have traveled a long distance before arriving in your kitchen. Farm-to-fork fresh? Unlikely. In spite of that, each offers a surprising array of "healthy" benefits.

- Familiarity
- Convenience

- Portability
- Well-portioned
- Flavorful

We can't ignore the fact—there's a strong appeal to packaged and processed food. Though deciding what's acceptable is a personal decision. There are no established, universal rules that govern keto-land. There's no need to explain yourself (or feel self-conscious about your choices). DIRTY, LAZY, KETO is a prejudice-free zone. No one here will judge you.

KETO CANDYLAND

How dirty are you? We're going to play a game. Review the below list of household products. Ask yourself, *Would I eat or drink this? Is it important to me?* If the answer is yes, even on occasion, circle the item. There are no right or wrong answers for this activity.

- champagne
- Splenda (sucralose; sugar-free sweetener)
- shredded cheese
- spinach in a bag (pre-washed)
- whipped cream in a can
- fast-food burger (no bun)
- vodka
- peanut butter
- energy drink (sugar-free or low-carb)
- olives (can or jar)
- tuna fish (can or pouch)
- eggs (not cage-free)

- diet soda
- green beans (can or frozen)
- sugar-free gelatin
- monk fruit (sugar-free sweetener)
- ranch dressing
- wine (dry)
- malt beverage or hard seltzer (low-carb)
- frozen blueberries
- hot dog
- toothpaste (for real!)
- low-carb tortilla
- tequila
- pickles (jar)
- nonstick cooking spray
- strawberries (frozen)
- cheese crisps
- sugar-free sweetener
- sauvignon blanc
- salmon (farm-raised, not wild)
- riced cauliflower (frozen)
- sugar-free gum
- frozen chicken strips (unbreaded, frozen)
- gin
- protein bar (low-carb)
- mayonnaise
- hard candy (sugar-free)
- deli lunch meat
- bouillon cubes
- chardonnay
- flavored water enhancers

- salsa (can or jar)
- hamburger (ground, fresh, not grass-fed beef)
- ice cream (low-carb)
- pre-packaged salad
- rum
- jam or preserves (sugar-free)
- broth (canned)
- multivitamins
- beer (low-carb)
- protein powder (low-carb)
- "keto"-labeled bread
- merlot
- chicken breast (flash-frozen)
- flavored coffee
- pancake syrup (sugar-free)
- coffee creamer (sugar-free)
- tomatoes (canned)
- energy drink (sugar-free or low-carb)
- breakfast sausage
- whiskey
- protein drink or shake (low-carb)
- vegetable oil
- string cheese
- wasabi almonds
- cabernet sauvignon
- beef jerky
- salad dressing (readymade)
- nuts (single-portion packages)
- cognac
- frozen vegetables (low-carb)

- "keto"-labeled cookies
- "keto"-labeled chips
- pumpkin (canned)
- "keto"-labeled cereal
- Jell-O cups
- cocoa-dusted almonds
- pork rinds
- bourbon
- hamburger patty (premade)
- frozen dinner (low-carb)
- chocolate chips (sugar-free)
- spicy peanuts
- scotch

Count the number of items you circled. Any number above twenty means you're pretty comfortable eating (or drinking) dirty keto foods. *Terrific!* You're already acquainted. Any number under ten reveals you might be more conservative in this arena. *That's fine too.* No matter what the total, everyone's a winner today. Being *on* the DIRTY, LAZY, KETO scoreboard is really all that matters.

DIRTY KETO COMFORT

Let me explain. This activity was not meant to exhaustively capture all things "dirty." Rather, it was to prove a point. What's deemed dirty lies in the eye of the beholder. You're likely using many of these already (at least with the toothpaste, *I hope so*). I wanted you to see how normal these products are. I think we can all agree now that we're all a little bit "dirty." The real question becomes, then: Is there any room for more?

If you find yourself feeling uncomfortable, pause for a second and think this next part through. What's *really* stopping you from getting down and dirty on the keto diet? Preference or cost, I can understand. For many of us, though, it's embarrassment. The stigma! There are a lot of misconceptions about the "correct" way and the "wrong" way to lose weight, even in the keto community. We are brainwashed to think that farm-to-table-*ish* foods are *always* the superior choice, no matter the situation. There's a lot of righteousness and indignation surrounding this topic. I've witnessed heated arguments break out over the sanctity of mayonnaise, tofu, or a bag of shredded cheese—*That's NOT KETO!*

Who knew talking about groceries could be so exciting?

📢 **You are not a bad person for drinking Diet Coke.**

CARB CRISIS

There are untold incentives for including packaged products during the weight loss journey; I don't want you to miss out. Face any preconceived notions about dirty keto foods now, or they might get in the way later—perhaps in a pinch or during a craving—when you need them the most. There will be a time when doing something rash (like licking the dust off a Doritos chip, which I have done) might seem like a plausible idea. (Can you say rock bottom?) Going "off the rails" isn't unheard of. You might start making plans for a punitive egg fast (tomorrow, of course) to right the wrongs of an all-out carb bender. Sound familiar? Stop that nonsense. *Pleeeeazzzzeee.* Keep your dignity. Instead, study what DIRTY, LAZY, KETO brings to the table. A backup plan.

> ⚠️ **What will happen when your appetite *DEMANDS* an "off-limit" food? Don't let a hankering cause you to spiral out of control. Establish an emergency plan *now*.**

Expect moments of weakness—anticipate them—we all know they exist. It's naïve to think we will always stay in control. Intellectually, we know there are other, more productive ways of dealing with our issues than turning toward high-carb foods for comfort (that's what Day 6 is all about). Nonetheless, even with the best intentions, most of us still make irrational decisions about food. *Don't let your fingers turn Cheeto orange.* Come see the value of a dirty keto alternative.

KETO COURTROOM

Thanks to DIRTY, LAZY, KETO, you've got options. Decide for yourself what's acceptable. We'll scrutinize the pros and cons of including dirty keto foods in your repertoire to prepare you better, starting by addressing common critical arguments.

DIRTY KETO DISADVANTAGES

1. CON: Dirty keto foods may lack any real nutritional value.

Yes, you called it right. Most junk food—not just keto-friendly snacks—is probably unhealthy. Packaged chips (even those cardboard-tasting cauliflower ones) aren't checking any boxes in the quality nutrition department. *Duh!* At any rate, is subsistence the sole reason we eat? Dirty keto foods, even "junk" foods, serve a well-meaning purpose. Emotional eating, celebrations, cravings. . . . If you determine that having a prepackaged snack is what stands between you and a carb bender blow-out, then I say GO FOR IT.

📣 **Poke through the contents of my purse, and you'll see how much I rely on dirty keto products. When I feel a burning desire to eat something sweet, I get desperate. This state of mind screams for a low-carb lifeline— one that I can dial up *FAST*. In situations like this, I find sugar-free candies (which contain a long list of chemical-sounding ingredients, none of which I can pronounce) are worth their weight in gold. No embarrassment here. I won't think twice about chomping an entire pack of gum in one sitting (one piece right after the next, spit out, and replaced as the sweetness starts to fade). And if I'm feeling extra-frantic, I might gnaw on a two-year-old chocolate protein bar, warped to an odd-looking banana shape from being smooshed at the bottom of my handbag. I won't think twice about using any of these options if it gets me through what feels like a life-or-death sugar craving.**

2. CON: Dirty keto foods may contain chemicals that could have a lasting effect on our overall health.

Correct-a-mungo. No one will argue otherwise! Commercially processed foods, even salad in a bag, likely contain ingredients (like preservatives) we don't fully understand. Now, is that a deal breaker? Strict keto says it is. I beg to differ. The convenience these foods offer—the ease with which they help us stay on track—for some outweighs any potential problems. You'll have to ask yourself whether it's justifiable or not. My opinion, not that you'll be shocked, is a resounding *YES*. They make keto *extra easy*.

> 👣 **I'm going to keep it real. I haven't cut up a head of lettuce since 1985.**

I like to think of dirty keto foods as taking out a student loan. No one likes the idea of being in debt. Be that as it may, if you need the help, they're a necessary evil, a means to a worthwhile end. Are there calculated risks involved? You bet. But at least in my mind, they are equally worth pursuing.

Whether to allow sugar-free sweeteners, preservatives, or chemicals in your keto foods is a personal choice. (I support you either way.)

3. CON: Specialty keto products are often expensive and hard to find.

Absolutely. I imagine some of the products described in this section are not for sale where you live. Does that mean you can't "do keto"? Definitely not! Travel-sized pouches of nuts may not be stocked at your grocery store (such a boring example, but someone wrote me a *looooooong* letter about this—*It just isn't fair!*), although that's not the point. Nuts (sold in a pouch) will not make or break your weight loss efforts;[68] be honest. Some-

---

68. Dear grumpy person worried about the availability of packaged nuts . . . what's stopping you from doling out portions of almonds into small containers yourself?

times you'll have to figure out how to make snack-size food all on your own.

Lacking access to keto junk food is not a deal-breaker. These foods are entirely unnecessary for losing weight. No one *needs* a low-carb ice cream bar, sugar-free cookie, or an eight-dollar box of keto cereal. These are *luxury* products—delightful to try, maybe (if you can find or afford them), but *NOT* a must-have.

Are these items not sold in your community? That's probably a blessing! Keep your money in your pocketbook and bite your tongue. Hold back any complaints (I'm covering up my ears). People from around the world have lost weight with DIRTY, LAZY, KETO[69] eating bona fide foods like chicken, butter, broccoli . . . (not "keto"-labeled chips!). Packaged products like those listed below are *not* a necessity.

COMMERCIAL KETO

Premade desserts: ice cream, cake, cookies, chocolates, candy

Breakfast treats: cereal, granola, baked goods, frozen waffles

Quick-fix mixes: muffin, cake, biscuit, mug cake, pancake

Substitution bread: tortillas, sandwich bread, rolls

Convenience-store foods: chips, protein bars

Syrups: pancake, honey, coffee flavors, chocolate

Sauces: barbecue, dips, marinades

Spreads: jam, preserves, chocolate

Specialty fats: MCT oil, avocado oil, flavored oil, grass-fed Irish butter

Additives: Himalayan pink salt, amino acid supplements, apple cider vinegar

---

69. Shout-out to *The DIRTY, LAZY, KETO: No Time to Cook Cookbook* translated and published in the Czech Republic!

4. CON: Dirty keto foods will "mess up" your weight loss.

Yes and no. Some of the ingredients found inside dirty keto foods can cause your weight to fluctuate—and in some cases, substantially. Whoa! Weight loss might become unstable (not to mention stressful). How will these foods affect you? Maybe not at all. The experience is not the same for everyone.

> ⚠ I personally experience a fleeting weight gain after consuming certain foods (almond flour, chia seeds, Carbquik, too many sugar alcohols). *I sometimes stay off the scale for a couple of days, so the change doesn't upset me.* Are you okay with this uncertainty? It's something to think about.

You'll have to do some research to figure out how dirty keto foods affect your body. As for consuming sugar-free sweeteners, everyone's metabolism reacts uniquely. Some folks don't fare well (stomach upset, flatulence, diarrhea, headache), while others continue to bob right along on their merry way. Indigestion isn't a rite of passage in keto-land, but the potential to have an adverse response is there.

"CORRECT" KETO SWEETENER

There's a lot of pressure to choose the "correct" keto sweetener. This one is natural. That one is not! Despite the rumors, there is no clear-cut answer here. What becomes too sweet to one person leaves another wanting more. Finding an acceptable sugar substitute is up to you. Availability, cost, tolerance, flavor—everyone has different expectations. All must be considered. Don't give up easily. With such a wide variety of styles and brands to choose from, keep trying them on for size until you find your right fit.

- Allulose (Sugar in the Raw)
- aspartame (Equal)
- monk fruit (Lakanto, Swerve)
- saccharin (Sweet'N Low)
- Stevia (Truvia)
- sucralose (Splenda)

📢 **What's the best tasting sugar-free sweetener? The one *you* like (and can tolerate). *Seriously!* Ignore the hype (and know-it-alls) and instead listen to your palate. There are plenty of options on the market for you to choose from.**

KETO CATCH-22

Dirty keto foods *can* wreak havoc, both physically and emotionally, when you step on the scale. Ironic, don't you think? The foods you thought were helping you somehow backfire. You may have thought you were doing everything right while your weight is much higher than expected. That's not fair. *Is it an actual gain?* (I guess it depends on how much low-carb ice cream you ate. A half-cup serving size, *really?*) It becomes a game of wait and see.

The not-knowing part and having to remain patient is anxiety-producing. Not everyone can handle this stress. For some, seeing an unexpected weight gain (even one that doesn't last) leads to hysteria (and maybe a regretful knee-jerk response to reverse it). Anticipating how you'll react is worth deliberation. You don't want to sabotage yourself. Take all of this into account as you develop your game plan.

5. CON: Dirty keto foods provoke you to overeat.

Possibly. When abused, high-calorie dirty keto "junk" foods can lead to a fiasco—weight gain is just the start. For some, taking "just a bite" triggers an inconsolable desire for more (and more, and MORE!). *Overeating, obsession, hoarding . . .* Destructive behaviors from the past could potentially resurface and escalate. Knowing this could happen, it's understandable to feel hesitant. Why tempt fate? If you have a history with a particular type of food (ice cream or chips come to mind), starting in again with a low-carb replacement might not be worth it.

6. CON: Once you get in the habit of using a dirty keto crutch, it's hard to stop.

Not necessarily. If developing a crutch is something you're worried about, do yourself a favor, and proceed cautiously at first. *Go slow.*

Will a substitution food "feed the habit" (making it harder to change an underlying behavior)? Potentially. Behavior is hard to predict. Some do well with small servings or periodic use. For these folks, dirty foods like keto bread or low-carb tortillas serve an admirable purpose. Such products can be beneficial, especially for newbies. They can be used occasionally or even as a stopgap without repercussion.

Not all substitution foods are created equal. For some, they can perpetuate old habits (which might be better to avoid). Keto-style waffles, French toast, pancakes *every day* for breakfast? Hmmm. I bet you see where I'm going with this. Be careful when introducing replacement versions of foods like this into your diet. If a problem arises, take swift action to correct it—if needed, ask for help.

CAUTIONARY KETO

Circle any foods that might create a dilemma for you. Did I miss something? Add them to the list.

- sweets (of any kind)
- ice cream (low-carb)
- sugar-free candy
- baked goods or desserts (low-carb)
- chaffle
- mug cake (low-carb)
- keto granola or cereal
- sugar-free chocolate
- specialty coffee drinks *(But they're sugar-free!)*
- heavy whipping cream
- fat bombs
- bread (low-carb); sliced bread, biscuits, breadsticks
- keto chips or crackers
- beef jerky
- pepperoni
- cheese
- peanut butter
- hummus

- pork rinds
- pizza (low-carb)

If you sense something might be wrong, *it probably is!* Your intuition is trying to tell you something. Listen closely. Internal alerts can prevent a trainwreck from happening. Be on the lookout for warning signs. Start by asking yourself these introspective questions:

- Do you have difficulty stopping when eating the food?
- Do you feel dependent on the food?
- Does the food cause you to exhibit undesirable behaviors (hoarding, overeating, obsessing)?

Ignoring a potential problem will only make it worse. Can you throw the food away or put some distance between you? At the very least, decide not to rebuy it.

> ⚠️ **Even though I sometimes get wild and crazy by topping my morning yogurt with sugar-free chocolate chips (once I open the bag, all bets are off!), I don't judge myself for moments of lost control *or pretend they won't happen*.**

KETO CONUNDRUM

There is no right or wrong answer for how best to handle "high-risk" foods. What works for one person may not be practical for someone else. Play with your options. Don't be afraid to try out-of-the-box solutions. If a strategy doesn't work, move on. Try something else (don't quit!). Here are some creative approaches for managing temptation.

🔊 I *love* low-carb desserts. So much so that I can't stop after just one (or two, okay . . . *three*) or more servings (some days, maybe the whole recipe). I know my limits! I can only handle making "treats" on an *infrequent* basis. Even then, to stop myself from going overboard, I use some creative maneuvers (they may not work for everyone). I immediately divide the finished recipe into several small containers and store them right away. "Hiding" the desserts (from myself, mind you) toward the bottom of my freezer (and covered up with other food) distracts me just long enough to forget about them. Is this song and dance ludicrous? You know it! *(Don't care tho.)* The extra effort doesn't bother me in the least. *Out of sight, out of mind.* I stop obsessing about having another. That's a win! I get to enjoy special treats occasionally, and more important, I do so on my terms.

TRICK TEMPTATION

Strategy	Explanation & Example
Break up for good.	Don't keep risky foods in the house. Notify the family—these foods are a no-go! For me, this means Doritos. Even hearing that word makes my mouth water!
Up high and hard-to-reach.	Relocate foods you want to avoid to an inconvenient location. I keep diet soda in the garage (unrefrigerated) to encourage myself to drink more water.

Forget about it.	Out-of-sight, out-of-mind. Strategically organize fridge/pantry shelves so tempting foods are tucked away. Look at the very bottom of my freezer to find my stash of low-carb desserts.
Accept an alternative.	Wholeheartedly embrace a satisfying substitute. Sugar-free cocktail? Cheers to that!
Delay, delay, delay.	When expected to provide a sugary treat (e.g., Halloween candy), purchase at the last second (and keep in the car).
A teensy tiny bit.	Invest in portion control. Individually wrapped ice cream bars, for instance, might be a better option than pints (where it's easy to go overboard).
Quality, not quantity.	Mindfully enjoy a small amount of the "good stuff." Gourmet chocolate and real whipped cream (from a can) come to mind.
Ruin it.	Can't avoid having this particular food around? Buy a style/variation that doesn't appeal to you. My story about Cheetos (coming up next) explains this point.

It's possible to outwit temptation. My kids adore Cheetos. Unfortunately, so do I! To avoid causing them to have emotional trauma from going without (kidding!), I buy them Flamin' Hot Cheetos (which is a flavor that doesn't interest me in the least).

Question dirty keto foods. That's part of the process! You won't be able to make a fair assessment about dirty keto foods, though, until you hear both sides. Study their positive attributes, too. Take into account all perspectives before hatching your personal plan. Are dirty keto foods worth the hassle? Only you can decide.

ADVANTAGES OF PLAYING DIRTY

1. PRO: A dirty keto product switcheroo is the path of least resistance.

A low-carb imitation exists for every food out there. It doesn't matter if you're itching for something salty or sweet, exotic or mundane; you can bet there's a keto clone available. Swapping out a high-carb food or drink with a similar keto-friendly version is a highly effective way to tame your appetites (without the high-carb backlash). It's a speedy, practical solution. Less painful too.

Changing up a morning coffee routine illustrates this concept nicely. Say you've spent the past forty years religiously drinking coffee with 2% milk and a spoonful of sugar. Would you be okay with suddenly drinking it black? Doubt it. *Err. Don't mess with mama's coffee.* That idea is destined to flop.

Now consider the switcheroo method. What if you used a deluxe sugar-free creamer in place of milk and sugar? (They come in fun flavors!) Or swap the low-fat milk for heavy whipping cream, and in lieu of table sugar, a sugar-free sweetener of your choice. Both have the same desired outcome—cutting carbs. But does one feel more sensible? With product substitutions, you won't have to turn your whole world (or at least your morning) upside down.

While this advice for weight loss may seem to go against conventional wisdom, at the same time, it works. *You* don't always have to be the one who changes. Try going about this backward. Change the food first, and see what happens. I know this won't work for every situation, but sometimes, taking the path of least resistance is more tolerable. *Swap out the food first and work on changing behaviors later.*

Are you hip to the legendary "bulletproof" coffee? Don't be scared by the aggressive name. It's just coffee with a bit of fat mixed in.

KETO COFFEE BREAK

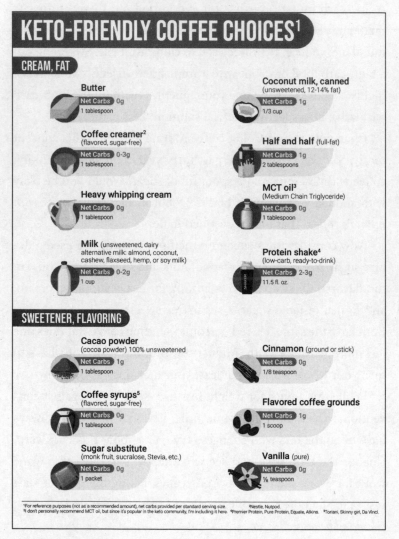

KETO-FRIENDLY COFFEE CHOICES[1]

CREAM, FAT

Butter
Net Carbs 0g
1 tablespoon

Coconut milk, canned
(unsweetened, 12-14% fat)
Net Carbs 1g
1/3 cup

Coffee creamer[2]
(flavored, sugar-free)
Net Carbs 0-3g
1 tablespoon

Half and half (full-fat)
Net Carbs 1g
2 tablespoons

Heavy whipping cream
Net Carbs 0g
1 tablespoon

MCT oil[3]
(Medium Chain Triglyceride)
Net Carbs 0g
1 tablespoon

Milk (unsweetened, dairy
alternative milk: almond, coconut,
cashew, flaxseed, hemp, or soy milk)
Net Carbs 0-2g
1 cup

Protein shake[4]
(low-carb, ready-to-drink)
Net Carbs 2-3g
11.5 fl. oz.

SWEETENER, FLAVORING

Cacao powder
(cocoa powder) 100% unsweetened
Net Carbs 1g
1 tablespoon

Cinnamon (ground or stick)
Net Carbs 0g
1/8 teaspoon

Coffee syrups[5]
(flavored, sugar-free)
Net Carbs 0g
1 tablespoon

Flavored coffee grounds
Net Carbs 1g
1 scoop

Sugar substitute
(monk fruit, sucralose, Stevia, etc.)
Net Carbs 0g
1 packet

Vanilla (pure)
Net Carbs 0g
1/8 teaspoon

[1]For reference purposes (not as a recommended amount), net carbs provided per standard serving size.   [2]Nestle, Nutpod.
[3]I don't personally recommend MCT oil, but since it's popular in the keto community, I'm including it here.   [4]Premier Protein, Pure Protein, Equate, Atkins.   [5]Torani, Skinny girl, Da Vinci.

2. PRO: With so many dirty keto foods at your disposal, you'll never need to go cold turkey.

Dirty keto foods can serve as a stopgap as you wean yourself off high-carb foods. Pasta comes to mind here. Newbies might try low-carb shirataki noodles[70] or Palmini noodles (from heart of palm) before moving on to a more affordable solution like zoodles (zucchini noodles). Nothing is wrong with using transitional products for longer (even permanently). If you feel the food is a stipulation for your success, it's worth the added effort or expense to keep it on hand. Does it interfere with your daily allotment of net carbs? No, you say. Then why not. Have at it.

> You don't have to jump into the deep end if you're not feeling confident. It's okay to take your time. Think of dirty keto foods like a pair of "floaties." They can help keep you buoyant as you learn to swim independently.

TRANSITION TIME
- sandwich bread (low-carb)
- tortillas (low-carb)
- shirataki noodles
- cheese taco shells
- ice cream (low-carb)
- keto cereal
- Carbquik Baking Mix

---

70. Pasta Zero, Miracle Noodle, and Wonder Noodles.

3. PRO: Emotionally, dirty keto foods can help you feel like you're not missing out.

Think back to the many diets you've tried (oh, jeez, for me, this could take a while). Did a compulsion for something "naughty" ever lead you astray? Taboo foods don't have to be our downfall any longer. A dirty keto substitute can prevent that from happening. They can help ward off feelings of deprivation or anger about "going without." For many, this is the *KEY*. No more "I'm on a diet" blues!

📢 **We eat for a variety of reasons beyond hunger; I eat when I'm feeling up (or down), excited, and bored. Will that behavior change anytime soon? Probably not. I don't care what people say (the criticism!). I'm fairly set in my ways.**

You don't have to miss out on familiar favorites. Avoid the FOMO! Find or arrange a keto-friendly substitute.

KETO COPYCATS

High-Carb Comfort Food	Low-Carb Substitute
Mashed potatoes and gravy	Mashed cauliflower and gravy
Spaghetti	Meat sauce over zoodles (zucchini noodles)
Waffle	Chaffle (cheese waffle)
Macaroni and cheese	Cauliflower with cheese
Lasagna	Eggplant lasagna
Milkshake	Protein smoothie

French fries	Asparagus fries
Chicken noodle soup	Broccoli cheese soup
Pizza	Meat-crusted pizza
Fried chicken	Fried chicken (low-carb coating)
Cheeseburger	Bunless cheeseburger
Tacos	Taco salad
Fried rice	Fried cauliflower rice
Enchiladas	Enchiladas made with egg wraps

 Creating copycat recipes is one of my passions. The more challenging, the better!

4. PRO: Desire something sweet? You can handle it.

A world-class sweet tooth doesn't have to be your downfall. Whether with a store-bought product or a low-carb recipe whipped up at home, you'll be able to handle any urges that come your way. Finding the perfect substitute is part of the fun. (Should we call it homework?) It's all about preparedness. When the sugar monster rears its ugly head, you'll want to have your low-carb harpoon locked and loaded. Get an immediate response plan in place—now.

CURB KETO CRAVINGS

Low-carb, sugar-free treats to satisfy a sweet tooth? Let's brainstorm.

- berries (strawberries, raspberries, blueberries, blackberries)
- coconut (unsweetened, shredded)
- sugar-free flavored gelatin

- hard candy (sugar-free)
- mug cake (low-carb)
- protein bar (low-carb)
- whipped cream (from a can)
- ice cream (low-carb)
- Cool Whip topping (try it frozen!)
- sugar-free chocolate bar
- cacao, 85 to 92% chocolate
- chocolate chips (sugar-free)
- peanut butter or nut butter
- herbal tea with heavy whipping cream and sugar-free sweetener
- low-carb smoothie
- coffee with sugar-free sweetener or sugar-free flavored syrup
- low-carb "milk" shake
- diet soda
- water with sugar-free flavor enhancer

Lately, my go-to snack for when I want something sweet is a bowl of sliced cucumbers (sprinkled with white distilled vinegar, sugar-free sweetener, and full-fat feta cheese). An off-the-wall combination for sure, but, at least for my palate, super tasty!

5. PRO: Dirty keto food options can help you fly under the radar.

Losing weight is personal. You don't have to share your weight loss journey with anyone if you don't want to. Talking about your diet can feel embarrassing and shameful, especially in a public setting like a restaurant. I put this in a category called "Nunya Business."[71] You might prefer to avoid drawing unnecessary attention to yourself by ordering verbatim off the menu—no special requests or modifications—just like everybody else. (No "diet" food for me!) With dirty keto foods, there are plenty of standard options. You can meet up with a friend for drinks or have a fast food (bunless) burger without being nervous (or falling off the wagon). Capitalize on these stealth maneuvers to keep your weight loss mission private.

OPERATION COVERT KETO

- Research the restaurant beforehand to determine what you'd like to order. Menus are often online (check the location's website or social review sites like Yelp). Call the restaurant to ask questions if needed.
- Order an appetizer (smaller portion).
- Investigate the a la carte (sides) section of the menu.
- Choose a standalone entree (without modifications) like a chef's salad with Diet Coke or ham and cheese omelet with coffee.
- Use the app to order (and make silent specifications).

📢 On a recent trip to Disneyland, I practiced ordering meals using their official park app. So convenient! Menu ingredients are listed in detail, which guided me to make better decisions. Additionally, I was able to order smaller portion sizes for myself from the children's menu (I'm a kid at heart, does that count?).

---

71. You've been warned. Nunya Business is none of your business!

6. PRO: Keto innovations keep daily life novel and fun.

Stumbling upon a new low-carb food option can be exciting—motivating even! I'm not talking about "keto"-advertised products (too obvious). I skip over those and hunt for "big game" within the regular food aisles. I scour random nutrition labels hoping to track down new keto-friendly foods. (If you tease me, I won't share what I found.)

SUPERMARKET SURPRISES

- affordable pasta sauce (no sugar added)[72]
- peeled hard-boiled eggs (could I be any lazier?)
- poke (seafood counter)
- prefab kebabs (raw meat counter)
- thin cuts of meat (they cook in less time)
- Indian-style simmer sauce (when added to chicken, it's just like takeout)
- frozen riced cauliflower (who has time to grate it themselves?)
- green beans sold in pre-packaged, microwavable packages for lunches
- travel-sized snacks that help with portion control (olives, nuts, cheese crisps)
- personal-sized guacamole cups
- stuffed mushrooms from the deli
- nut butter (no sugar added) in single-serving squeezable pouches

---

72. Hunt's 100% Natural Tomato Sauce, Hunt's Pasta Sauce (No Added Sugar).

- rotisserie chicken[73]
- celery stalks (pre-washed, pre-cut)
- low-carb yogurts (new brands pop up weekly!)
- freshly made jalapeño poppers (not breaded) from the deli
- portable *sealed* salads (chef, Caesar) that include dressing and utensils
- frozen avocado chunks (so convenient for making smoothies)

After navigating through Day 6, where did you land? At the very least, I hope you have broadened your definition of dirty keto. I don't want you feeling pressured to use products you aren't comfortable with. But at the same time, I hope you're now evaluating options with an open mind. Remember, you won't be going in blind as you trial new products as we've already examined potential complications with great care. That's not to say your journey won't get messy here and there as you establish personal limits. In the end, let me assure you, it will all have been worth it.

KETO CONVICTION

Dirty keto foods make weight loss attainable. They provide shortcuts, convenience, and quash cravings. I can bank on them to get me out of a pinch. Meal planning is a snap with semi-prepped ingredients. Saving time while having fun? Dirty keto foods make this way of life enjoyable. It's an *Extra Easy Keto* life I can do *for-evah*.

---

73. Costco's 3-pound rotisserie chickens and famous hot dog/soda combination (toss the bun) have sold at a fixed price, well below market, for over a decade. What a steal!

📢 **How ironic. Dirty keto foods might be the glue holding this all together.**

Vow to lose weight differently this time. Take a stand. Decide for yourself what constitutes optimal eating. Practice listening to your gut and become liberated. *You know more than you think you do.*

Don't let society's narrow definition of healthiness stop you from experiencing what dirty keto foods have to offer. Maybe you have a sweet tooth? Stop fighting it. There is no shame in enjoying a low-carb beer or sugar-free dessert while losing weight. It's perfectly acceptable to cut corners with meal prep too. A home-cooked meal tastes just as marvelous (if not better) when prepared in half the time, wouldn't you agree? When used wisely, dirty keto foods can be your surefire weapon in this battle. Come prepared to the weight loss arena. Strengthen yourself with the most unsuspecting tool of all: *options.*

📋 **Day 6 Marching Orders**

1. *Define "dirty keto." Has your opinion about it changed? Explain.*
2. *Make a list of your must-have and must-avoid dirty keto foods. What is your reasoning?*
3. *Talk about foods to be wary around. How will you know if a particular dirty keto food becomes a problem? Come up with a plan.*

DAY 7: ALL IN

We've been on quite a journey together. Can you believe it's only been a week? If you haven't been implementing changes (establishing healthy habit rituals, meal-planning with the Big Three), now is the time to begin. Not next Monday, not January, *NOT* after your vacation. *Today.* If your gut is telling you to wait, push back. Coach yourself through the urge to stall. It's okay to start before you feel 100% confident. Fake it 'til you make it, if need be. No one expects you to do DIRTY, LAZY, KETO *perfectly* (is that even a thing?). Be vulnerable. Remember, there is no punishment for falling short.

> ⚠️ **Stomp out the urge to do keto flawlessly. Perfectionism is a breeding ground for burnout, anxiety, depression, and procrastination.**

KETO KARMA

You have everything you need to be successful on keto. Which resource will you lean on the most? No, it's not the grocery list (good guess, though). It's actually something you've had with you all along. I hope this doesn't sound cheesy (you know I take my dairy seriously), but here goes anyway. It's your attitude! Whether you think you can or can't, you're *totally* right.

Believing in yourself is *EVERYTHING*.

Once you get in a positive frame of mind, making decisions about what to eat *and* when to eat it will become part of your DNA.

Not completely convinced? To remove any lingering doubt you might have (it's okay to be nervous!), today we'll build a step-by-step meal plan to get you through the first week. I'll help you get the ball rolling. Day 7 includes a week's worth of *Extra Easy Keto* meal and snack suggestions. Before peeking at my ideas, try to brainstorm thoughts of your own. Here is some advice to keep in mind.

KETO CRUNCH TIME

1. Eat foods you like.
2. It's okay to replay favorite meals or snacks.
3. Less is more. Fewer ingredients set the stage for accuracy.
4. Avoid lopsided meals. Eat throughout the day to help ward off hunger pains and maintain energy levels.
5. Don't forget drinks.
6. Plan for low-carb treats (notice I didn't say cheating).
7. Take ownership of your game plan; enjoy yourself.

The objective for Day 7 is for you to complete a very "eatable" 7-day menu that reflects your preferences, not mine. *You know more than you think you do!* Use the provided blank template on the next page as a framework. If you become tempted to skip this project (and search out someone else's "official" keto meal plan to follow), take a deep breath, place your right hand on a pack of bacon (LOL), and repeat this oath after me.

THE DLK COMMITMENT

I, (insert name), do solemnly swear to go all in with DIRTY, LAZY, KETO. Today, I wave goodbye to crash diets. I realize they are temporary Band-Aids that won't help me in the long run. I am capable of real change. My health is worth it! I promise to be patient with myself and stay positive. I know I can do this because you don't have to be perfect to be successful. This pledge is my DLK commitment.

MEAL MIX-N-MATCH

Need help starting? Get inspired by the assortment of DIRTY, LAZY, KETO meals and drinks described below. These are *not* recipes, only meal ideas.[74] (I include an ingredient breakdown as a teachable handy reference.) Net carb counts are per single serving (except where otherwise noted). Should you encounter any discrepancy between what's listed here and what you find in your kitchen, defer to the product in your hand.[75]

---

74. Take the omelet suggestion, for example. I share how mushrooms contain 2 grams net carbs per 1-cup serving—*that doesn't mean you should add a whole cup to your one-egg omelet!*

75. Manufacturers do not all use the same ingredients. Net carb counts can vary among competing brands. Your best bet is to look at the Nutrition Facts label of every food you eat.

CARB *Tracker*

	MON	TUE	WED	THU	FRI	SAT	SUN
DATE:							
BREAKFAST							
LUNCH							
DINNER							
SNACKS							
WATER	🥤🥤🥤🥤🥤🥤🥤🥤	🥤🥤🥤🥤🥤🥤🥤🥤	🥤🥤🥤🥤🥤🥤🥤🥤	🥤🥤🥤🥤🥤🥤🥤🥤	🥤🥤🥤🥤🥤🥤🥤🥤	🥤🥤🥤🥤🥤🥤🥤🥤	🥤🥤🥤🥤🥤🥤🥤🥤
NET CARBS:							

Weekly Weigh-In: _____   Today's Date: _____

Notes:

EXTRA EASY KETO BREAKFAST IDEAS

EGGS AND SAUSAGE

Eggs, 1g net carb per egg

Butter, 0g net carbs per tablespoon

Sausage, breakfast (varies by brand), estimated 0–2g net carbs per 2–3 links

SPINACH AND MUSHROOM OMELET

Eggs, 1g net carb per egg

Spinach (raw), 0g net carbs per cup

Mushrooms (raw, sliced), 2g net carbs per cup

Swiss cheese, 1g net carb per ounce

Butter, 0g net carbs per tablespoon

PROTEIN SMOOTHIE

Protein powder (sugar-free), 1g net carb per scoop

Milk (unsweetened, dairy alternative milk: almond, coconut, cashew, flaxseed, hemp, or soy milk), varies by
brand, estimated 0–2g net carbs per cup

Sugar substitute (monk fruit, sucralose, Stevia, etc.), 0g net
carbs per packet

Spinach (raw), 0g net carbs per cup

Blackberries, 6g net carb per cup

Ice, 0g net carbs per 8 ounces

BULLETPROOF COFFEE

Coffee (black), 0g net carbs per 8 fl. ounces

Heavy whipping cream, 0g net carbs per tablespoon

Sugar substitute (monk fruit, sucralose, Stevia, etc.), 0g net
carbs per packet

CINNAMON TOASTED YOGURT WITH WALNUTS

Yogurt (5% milkfat, Greek, strained, plain), 5g net carbs per
¾ cup

Sugar substitute (monk fruit, sucralose, Stevia, etc.), 0g net
carbs per packet

Vanilla (pure), 0g net carbs per ⅛ teaspoon

Cinnamon (ground or stick), 0g net carbs per ⅛ teaspoon

Walnut (halves and pieces), 2g net carbs per ounce

GRAB-AND-GO BREAKFAST

Egg (hard-boiled), 1g net carb per egg

Cheese (string), 1g net carb per ounce

Deli meat (varies by brand), estimated 1g net carb per 2 ounces

COTTAGE CHEESE WITH FRUIT

Cottage cheese, 4% milkfat, 5g net carbs per ½ cup

Blueberries,[76] 5g net carbs per ¼ cup

EXTRA EASY KETO LUNCH/DINNER IDEAS

CHICKEN CAESAR SALAD

Chicken, 0g net carbs per 4 ounces

Lettuce (romaine), 1g net carb per 1½ cups

Salad dressing (Caesar), 1g net carb per 2 tablespoons

Parmesan cheese (grated), 1g net carb per ounce

PESTO SHRIMP WITH ZUCCHINI NOODLES (ZOODLES)

Shrimp, 0g net carbs per 3 ounces

Zucchini (raw), 1g net carb per cup

Pesto (varies by brand), estimated 1–5g net carbs per ¼ cup

Parmesan cheese (grated), 1g net carb per ounce

FAJITA CHICKEN STRIPS WITH GREEN BELL PEPPERS

Chicken, 0g net carbs per 4 ounces

Bell pepper (green), sliced, 4g net carbs per cup

Oil, 0g net carbs per tablespoon

Taco seasoning,[77] 3–4g net carbs per 2 teaspoons

---

76. Blueberries have 18 grams net carbs for the "standard" 1 cup serving.

77. Serving size for 1 pound meat (approximately 12 tacos).

STEAK AND GREEN BEANS

Steak, 0g net carbs per 3 ounces

Green beans (string), 4g net carbs per cup

Butter, 0g net carbs per tablespoon

BUNLESS BURGER TOPPED WITH SAUTEED MUSHROOMS AND GORGONZOLA CHEESE

Hamburger patty, 0g net carbs per 4 ounces

Mushrooms (raw), sliced, 2g net carbs per cup

Gorgonzola cheese, 1g net carb per ounce

TURKEY TACO BOATS

Ground turkey, 0g net carbs per 3 ounces

Taco seasoning,[78] 3–4g net carbs per 2 teaspoons

Lettuce (romaine), 0g net carbs per 3 leaves

Cheddar cheese, 1g net carb per ounce

Sour cream (full-fat), 1g net carb per 2 tablespoons

Olives (black), 1g net carb per 2 large olives

Tomato, 5g net carbs per medium tomato

Avocado, 1g net carb per ⅓ of a medium avocado

CATFISH AND COLLARD GREENS

Seafood, 0g net carbs per 3 ounces

Oil, 0g net carbs per tablespoon

Creole seasoning mix, 0g net carbs per ¼ teaspoon

Collard greens (cooked), 3g net carbs per cup

Butter, 0g net carbs per tablespoon

---

78. Serving size for 1 pound meat (approximately 12 tacos).

EXTRA EASY KETO SNACK IDEAS

GUACAMOLE

Avocado, 1g net carb per ⅓ of a medium avocado

Lime juice, 0g net carbs per teaspoon, 1g net carb per tablespoon

Garlic (minced), 1g net carb per teaspoon

Cilantro (fresh, chopped), 0g net carbs per tablespoon

CELERY AND CREAM CHEESE

Celery, 1g net carb per cup

Cream cheese, full-fat, 1–2g net carbs per ounce

TRAIL MIX

Almonds, 3g net carbs per ounce

Chocolate chips (sugar-free, sweetened with monk fruit[79]), 1g net carb per 60 chips (14 grams)

Coconut (unsweetened, shredded) 2g net carbs per 2 tablespoons

BROCCOLI FLORETS WITH RANCH DRESSING

Broccoli (fresh), 4g net carbs per cup

Salad dressing (ranch), 1g net carb per 2 tablespoons

BACON-WRAPPED ASPARAGUS

Asparagus, 2g net carbs per cup

Bacon (unflavored), 0g net carbs per 2 cooked slices

---

79. ChocZero, Lakanto.

SIDE SALAD

Salad greens (lettuce mix), 1g net carb per 2 cups

Tomatoes (cherry), 2g net carbs per 3 cherry tomatoes

Oil, 0g net carbs per tablespoon

Vinegar, 0g net carbs per tablespoon

DEVILED EGGS

Egg, 1g net carb per egg

Mayonnaise (full-fat), 0g net carbs per tablespoon

Vinegar (plain white), 0g net carbs per tablespoon

Mustard (yellow), 0g net carbs per teaspoon

EXTRA EASY KETO DESSERT IDEAS

STRAWBERRIES WITH WHIPPED CREAM

Strawberries (whole), 8g net carbs per cup

Sugar substitute (monk fruit, sucralose, Stevia, etc.), 0g net
carbs per packet

Whipped dairy topping in a can (regular), 1g net carb per
2 tablespoons

SUGAR-FREE JELL-O SUNDAE

Gelatin (sugar-free, any flavor), 0g net carbs per ½ cup prepared

Sour cream (full-fat), 1g net carb per 2 tablespoons

Peanuts (roasted, salted), 3g net carbs per ounce

CHOCOLATE CHIP YOGURT

Yogurt (5% milkfat, Greek, strained, plain), 5g net carbs per ¾ cup

Sugar substitute (monk fruit, sucralose, Stevia, etc.), 0g net carbs per packet

Vanilla (pure), 0g net carbs per ⅛ teaspoon

Chocolate chips (sugar-free, sweetened with monk fruit[80]), 1g net carb per 60 chips (14 grams)

RASPBERRIES AND CREAM

Raspberries, 7g net carbs per cup

Heavy whipping cream, 0g net carbs per tablespoon

Sugar substitute (monk fruit, sucralose, Stevia, etc.), 0g net carbs per packet

BITE OF CHOCOLATE

Cacao, 92% chocolate, 6g net carbs per 3 pieces (34 grams)

CHOCOLATE SHAKE

Milk (unsweetened, dairy alternative milk: almond), 1g net carb per cup

Avocado, 1g net carb per ⅓ of a medium avocado

Cacao powder (cocoa powder), 100% unsweetened, 1g net carb per tablespoon

Sugar substitute (monk fruit, sucralose, Stevia, etc.), 0g net carbs per packet

Vanilla (pure), 0g net carbs per ⅛ teaspoon

Ice, 0g net carbs per cup

---

80. ChocZero, Lakanto, Lily's Sweets.

SUGAR-FREE CANDY

Hard candy (sugar-free), varies by brand, estimated 0–1g net carbs per 4–6 pieces

EXTRA EASY KETO DRINK[01] IDEAS

Beer (low-carb),[82] varies by brand, estimated 3–5g net carbs per 12 fl. ounces

Champagne, 1g net carb per 5 fl. ounces

Chardonnay, 3g net carbs per 5 fl. ounces

Coffee (black), 0g net carbs per 8 fl. ounces

Diet soda, 0g net carbs per 8 fl. ounces

Electrolyte-enhanced water,[83] 0g net carbs per 8 fl. ounces

Energy drinks (sugar-free or low-carb),[84] 0–3g net carbs per 8 fl. ounces

Flavored drink enhancers (sugar-free), 0–3g net carbs per serving[85]

Liquor (unflavored hard alcohol),[86] 0g net carbs per 1.5 fl. oz.

Malt beverages (low-carb), varies by brand,[87] estimated 1–5g net carbs per 12 fl. ounces

Milk (unsweetened, dairy alternative milk: almond, coconut,

---

81. A variety of zero-carb or low-carb drink ideas are provided here for your reference (other than water, none of these drinks are "required").

82. Busch Light, Corona Premier, Michelob Ultra, Miller Lite, Natural Light.

83. MiO, Propel, Smartwater.

84. Bang, Sugar-free Monster, Sugar-free Red Bull.

85. Serving sizes vary among brands.

86. Brandy, gin, rum, sake, tequila, vodka, whiskey.

87. Bon & Viv, Henry's, Smirnoff, Truly, White Claw.

cashew, flaxseed, hemp, or soy milk), varies by brand, estimated 0–2g net carbs per cup

Mineral water or naturally flavored water (sugar-free), 0g net carbs per 8 fl. ounces

Red wine (pinot noir), 3g net carbs per 5 fl. ounces

Seltzer water (sugar-free), 0g net carbs per 8 fl. ounces

Soda water (sugar-free), 0g net carbs per 8 fl. ounces

Sports drink (sugar-free),[88] 0–1g net carb per 8 fl. ounces

Tea (unsweetened, sugar-free: herbal, black, green), 0g net carbs per 8 fl. ounces

Tonic water (sugar-free), 0g net carbs per 8 fl. ounces

Water (flat), 0g net carbs per 8 fl. ounces

White wine (sauvignon blanc), 3g net carbs per 5 fl. ounces

Wine (dry), 3–4g net carbs per 5 fl. ounces

BONUS MATERIAL: 10 *EXTRA EASY KETO* STARTER RECIPES

You're ready for the big leagues: making low-carb recipes from "scratch." (Don't be alarmed, I use the term "scratch" loosely!) Next, you'll find ten *Extra Easy Keto* recipes that span from sweets to snacks and even a full meal. Surely something here will tickle your fancy. What will you make first?

---

88. Gatorade Zero, Powerade Zero Sugar, Propel Zero Sugar Electrolyte Water Beverage.

CHILDHOOD CHICKEN NUGGETS WITH HONEY MUSTARD DIPPIN' SAUCE

Call me childish if you want to, but chicken nuggets are one of my favorite meals. There is something so whimsical about finger food! This crowd-pleasing recipe hits all the notes. Crispy "fried" chicken with a tangy dippin' sauce that's finger-licking good. You'll be thrilled how fast this meal comes together. Skip the drive-thru and plug in the air fryer instead.

Serves 2 (about 5 nuggets per serving)

Net carbs: 2g net carbs per serving

Prep time: 15 minutes

Cook time: 19 minutes

Nuggets
½ pound boneless, skinless chicken breasts, cut into 2 x 2-inch
    pieces (about 8–10 nuggets)

1 tablespoon vegetable oil

1 large egg

¼ cup grated Parmesan cheese

½ teaspoon ranch powder seasoning

Honey Mustard Dippin' Sauce
¼ cup full-fat mayonnaise

2 teaspoons yellow mustard

2 (1-gram) packets 0g net carb sweetener

⅛ teaspoon Worcestershire sauce

1. In a small bowl, evenly coat chicken with oil.

2. Arrange coated nuggets on your air fryer's crisper tray, making sure they are not touching. Cook 14 minutes at 400°F. Remove from air fryer. The nuggets should be partially cooked.

3. Set out 2 small bowls. In one bowl, whisk the egg. In the second bowl, combine the Parmesan cheese with ranch powder seasoning.

4. One at a time, dip the partially cooked nuggets into the egg mixture, shake off excess, then roll in the cheese mixture to coat evenly.

5. Return breaded nuggets to the crisper tray, making sure they are not touching. Cook 5 minutes at 400°F.

6. In a small bowl, combine all ingredients to make the Dippin' Sauce and stir until blended. Divide into 2 small serving bowls.

7. Remove nuggets from the air fryer and divide between two serving plates. Serve warm with a bowl of Dippin' Sauce on each plate.

Extra Easy Keto Tips & Options

Don't have an air fryer? *No biggie.* Place coated nuggets on a greased 9 x 9-inch baking dish and bake at 375°F until the internal temperature reaches at least 165°F, flipping halfway through.

Skip a step and get to the best part sooner (eating!). Ranch dressing (purchased from the grocery store) makes a delightful dipping sauce all on its own.

HOLLA JALAPEÑO POPPERS

Never throw away an "empty" jar of pickles. The juice that's left behind is chock full of flavor and electrolytes. Sip away—it can help ward off the "keto flu." I add this informal ingredient to all sorts of recipes (marinades, salad dressings) for flavor. Pickle juice gives these jalapeño poppers a delightful zing. Live a little!

Serves 4 (2 poppers per serving)
Net carbs: 2g net carbs per serving
Prep time: 10 minutes
Cook time: 10 minutes

4 ounces full-fat cream cheese, softened
1 tablespoon pickle juice
¼ cup shredded cheddar cheese
4 large jalapeños, halved, seeded, and deveined
8 strips no-sugar-added bacon

1. In a small bowl, combine the cream cheese, pickle juice, and cheddar cheese. Stir until blended.
2. Divide the cream cheese mixture evenly between jalapeño halves. Wrap one strip of bacon around each jalapeño.
3. Evenly spread jalapeños on the crisper tray of an air fryer and cook 8 to 10 minutes at 400°F. Serve warm.

Extra Easy Keto Tips & Options

In place of an air fryer, bake these jalapeños in a traditional oven at 400°F for 8 to 10 minutes (or until the bacon reaches the desired level of crispiness).

When preparing your jalapeños, I warn you to wear food-grade gloves (and maybe even a mask) for protection. Be sure to remove all seeds from inside the pepper—those are what make a jalapeño *hot, hot, hot!*

FORTUNATE CHICKEN FETTUCCINE ALFREDO

Some argue that Fettuccine Alfredo is the unhealthiest dish served in America. That's quite a statement! My keto-friendly version of this beloved favorite won't raise any eyebrows. Zucchini noodles, or "zoodles," replace traditional high-carb pasta in this dish. These aren't complicated or expensive to make, either. With a few snappy swipes of a hand-held julienne peeler, you'll have "fettuccine" created in no time.

Serves 2
Net carbs: 3g net carbs per serving
Prep time: 15 minutes
Cook time: 9 minutes

2 medium zucchinis
1 tablespoon olive oil
2 tablespoons unsalted butter
½ ounce full-fat cream cheese, softened
¼ cup heavy whipping cream
1 tablespoon grated Parmesan cheese
½ teaspoon garlic, minced
¼ teaspoon black ground pepper
¼ teaspoon salt
½ cup cooked rotisserie chicken, chopped

1. Using a julienne peeler, create "zoodles" by peeling the zucchini lengthwise in strips (skin can stay on).

2. Heat the oil in a medium skillet over medium heat. Add zoodles to the skillet and toss to coat with the oil. Cook 3 to 4 minutes, stirring often, until zoodles are tender. Remove from heat and set aside.

3. Melt the butter in a small saucepan over low heat. Add the remaining ingredients, except the chicken, and whisk until cheese is melted and a thick, uniform sauce forms (about 5 minutes). Gently fold in the chicken and zoodles to combine.

4. Divide evenly between 2 dinner plates. Serve warm.

Extra Easy Keto Tips & Options

Can you handle the heat? Sprinkle ⅛ teaspoon red pepper flakes into the sauce as it cooks.

Watch the sauce closely to prevent curdling. Double check (then triple check) the burner flame is turned low. Should a high heat misstep occur, try whisking in an additional teaspoon of heavy whipping cream.

Cooked shrimp can replace chicken in this recipe. Shrimp is a high-protein, low-carb keto favorite, with 0 grams net carbs per 3-ounce serving.

Don't feel like making sauce from scratch tonight? I won't tell. Substitute alfredo sauce purchased from the supermarket. *Shhh!* (Be sure to bury the "evidence" deep in the trash can.)

CAN'T-BEAT-IT BEANLESS CHILI

When folks are new to the low-carb community, they often obsess about beans. "HOW do you eat chili? What about the BEANS?" Let me reassure you, once traditional flavors are added to a recipe, like in this keto-friendly chili, you'll soon forget about those high-carb offenders. The texture and spices here invent a new comfort food favorite. The heat can't be beat!

Serves 4 (about ¾ cup per serving)

Net carbs: 4g net carbs per serving

Prep time: 20 minutes

Cook time: 36 minutes

½ pound 85% lean ground beef

⅛ teaspoon salt

¼ teaspoon ground black pepper, divided

1 tablespoon olive oil

2 tablespoons finely chopped green onion

½ cup chopped green bell pepper

½ cup chopped celery

1 cup thinly sliced mushrooms

1 teaspoon garlic, minced

1¾ cups vegetable broth

¾ cup tomato sauce (no sugar added)

1½ teaspoons chili powder

¼ teaspoon ground cumin

¼ teaspoon dried oregano

¼ teaspoon onion powder

1. In a large stock pot over medium heat, cook the beef 10 to 15 minutes, stirring regularly until browned. Season with salt and ⅛ teaspoon of the ground black pepper. Transfer meat to a large bowl (do not drain excess fat).

2. In the pot, heat olive oil over medium heat. Add the green onion, bell pepper, celery, and mushrooms. Saute 7 to 10 minutes until softened. Add garlic and stir until fragrant, about 30 seconds to 1 minute.

3. Add ground beef and remaining ingredients to the pot, along with remaining ⅛ teaspoon ground black pepper, and stir.

4. Cover pot and reduce heat to low. Let simmer 10 minutes.

5. Remove from heat and let cool uncovered. Divide evenly between 4 soup bowls and serve.

Extra Easy Keto Tips & Options

Serve topped with a sprinkle of shredded cheddar cheese.

Prefer less spice? Reduce chili powder to desired level of heat.

SPLENDID SPINACH SALAD WITH SALMON, GOAT CHEESE, & CANDIED WALNUTS

I'll try any recipe if it includes something candied—what about you? I often turn to strategies like this to make nutritious eating more bearable. I'll even tolerate eating spinach if there's a possibility my fork could pick up something delectable like goat cheese or a sweetened walnut. There's nothing wrong with using juvenile tactics like this. We've got to eat our veggies any way we can.

Serves 4 (¼ of the salad and 1 fillet per serving)
Net carbs: 1g net carb per serving
Prep time: 15 minutes
Cook time: 17 minutes

Salmon
 4 (3-ounce) salmon fillets, skin on
 1 tablespoon olive oil
 ¼ teaspoon salt, divided
 1 tablespoon unsalted butter, melted

Candied Nuts
 2 tablespoons unsalted butter
 3 tablespoons 0g net carb brown sugar substitute, divided
 ¼ teaspoon pure vanilla extract
 ¼ teaspoon cinnamon
 1 cup shelled walnuts, halves and pieces
 ⅛ teaspoon salt

Salad

8 cups spinach leaves

¼ cup sesame oil

2 tablespoons vinegar

8 (1-gram) packets 0g net carb sweetener

¼ cup full-fat goat cheese, crumbled

1. Brush all sides of salmon fillets with olive oil and rub with ⅛ teaspoon of the salt.
2. Evenly spread the fillets so they are not touching on an air fryer crisper tray. Cook 12 minutes at 400°F.
3. While still in crisper tray, evenly brush the tops of the fish with butter and sprinkle with remaining ⅛ teaspoon salt. Return the drawer to the air fryer and cook additional 2 minutes at 400°F. Remove from air fryer and set aside.
4. To make the candied nuts, in a small skillet over medium heat, melt 2 tablespoons butter. Add 2 tablespoons of the brown sugar substitute, vanilla, and cinnamon and stir, about 2 to 3 minutes. When the brown sugar substitute is dissolved, add walnuts. Use a silicone spatula to gently stir, turning over nuts until evenly coated. Remove from heat.
5. Transfer nut mixture to a parchment-lined dinner plate in a thin, even layer. When cool enough to touch, break apart into a crumble. Sprinkle with ⅛ teaspoon salt and remaining tablespoon of the brown sugar substitute. Set aside.
6. Add spinach to a large salad bowl.
7. In a small mixing bowl, make the salad dressing by whisking together sesame oil, vinegar, and sweetener. Pour over spinach and toss until leaves are evenly coated.

8. Divide salad between 4 serving plates. Top each with 1 salmon fillet. Sprinkle with equal amounts goat cheese and candied nuts. Serve immediately.

Extra Easy Keto Tips & Options

Substitute any low-carb nut here. Macadamia nuts or pecans would make an acceptable swap for walnuts.

Freeze leftover nut mixture (As if! It's doubtful there will be any extra.).

Not a fan of goat cheese? Try full-fat feta crumbles (or omit cheese altogether).

No air fryer—*really?* (Come on, you really need to think about getting one.) Cook fish on the stovetop instead: using a medium-sized frying pan over medium heat, fry fish in 1 tablespoon of butter for 3 to 5 minutes on each side until cooked.

Salmon does not have to be served warm. A chilled salmon fillet is also delicious.

NO RULES-ZA DEEP DISH PIZZA

Losing weight while eating pizza? Yessiree! Cut out the crust to cut back on carbs. This "deep dish" pizza holds up surprisingly well (though you will need to eat it with a fork—work with me, people). Since this dish is so delish, *I predict you'll crave seconds. Serve each slice with a generous side salad (romaine lettuce has 1 gram net carb per cup) as vegetables help us "slow our roll."*

Serves 4 (¼ pizza per serving)

Net carbs: 4g net carbs per serving

Prep time: 15 minutes

Cook time: 55 minutes

½ pound 93% lean ground beef

1 teaspoon Italian seasoning

1¼ cups shredded cheddar cheese, divided

⅛ teaspoon salt

½ cup no-sugar-added pasta sauce[89]

1 cup shredded whole-milk mozzarella cheese

8 pepperoni slices

1. Preheat oven to 375°F. Grease an 8 x 8 x 2-inch baking dish.
2. In a medium nonstick skillet over medium heat, cook beef for 10 to 15 minutes while stirring. Remove from heat and drain any excess fat.
3. Add Italian seasoning, 1 cup of the cheddar cheese, and salt to drained meat and stir until blended. Using a spatula, evenly press mixture into bottom of baking dish.

---

89. Consider Hunt's 100% Natural Tomato Sauce, Hunt's Pasta Sauce (No Sugar Added), or Rao's Homemade Pasta Sauce.

4. Evenly spread pasta sauce over meat mixture. Top with layer of mozzarella cheese.

5. Evenly sprinkle with remaining cheddar cheese then decorate with pepperoni.

6. Cover with foil and bake 30 minutes. Remove foil and bake 5 to 10 additional minutes until cheese begins to brown on top.

7. Cut into 4 slices and serve warm.

Extra Easy Keto Tips & Options

Feel free to customize your pizza toppings. Be sure to adjust the number of net carbs based on what you add to the meal. Here are some low-carb veggie suggestions (based on a 2-tablespoon serving, appropriate for this size pizza): chopped green onion, 1g net carb; sliced black olives, 1g net carb; sliced mushrooms, 0g net carbs; chopped tomato, 2g net carbs; sliced jalapeño (rings), 0g net carbs; chopped green bell pepper, 1g net carb; chopped broccoli, 1g net carb; spinach, 0g net carbs.

PRIZE-WINNING "POTATO" CUPS

Boring and predictable, potatoes are cheap, versatile, and effortless to cook. They're easy—I get it! But here's the deal. There are less starchy options available (e.g., a head of cauliflower) that can serve the same purpose. You'll never meet a more versatile low-carb vegetable! Once mashed (and mixed with something flavorful, like cream, bacon bits, and seasonings), a cauliflower side dish just might become a staple in your household, if not the most requested family favorite. This savory dish has a mouthfeel like potatoes and looks the part to boot. Bring it to your next social event and watch the tongues wag ("This ain't diet food!").

Serves 8 (about 3 per serving)

Net carbs: 3g net carbs per serving

Prep time: 20 minutes

Cook time: 60 minutes

1 tablespoon olive oil

1 cup water

1 large head of cauliflower, cut into ½- to 1-inch florets

3 large eggs, beaten

¼ cup heavy whipping cream

¼ teaspoon garlic, minced

¼ teaspoon salt

¼ teaspoon ground black pepper

3 tablespoons finely chopped green onion

1½ cups shredded cheddar cheese, divided

¼ cup bacon bits

1. Preheat oven to 350°F. Grease bottom and sides of 24 baking cups by brushing each with oil.

2. In a pressure cooker, insert trivet and add water and cauliflower. Lock the lid. Cook on pressure cooking setting at high pressure for 20 minutes. Release pressure and unlock lid.

3. Carefully remove trivet and add eggs, cream, garlic, salt, pepper, onion, and ½ cup of cheddar cheese. Using a hand mixer, blend thoroughly to combine (small lumps of cauliflower are fine).

4. Divide cauliflower mixture evenly between greased baking cups (approximately 3 tablespoons of mixture per cup).

5. Top each cup with bacon bits and remaining cheddar cheese.

6. Cover with foil and bake 35 to 40 minutes at 350°F, removing foil for the last 5 to 10 minutes of cook time to allow cheese to brown.

7. Let cool, then serve warm.

Extra Easy Keto Tips & Options

Serve with a dollop of full-fat sour cream on the side for dipping.

You're not alone if you find this twice-baked "potato" recipe has an air of breakfast to it. Perhaps it makes you think about biscuits or morning hash browns? Serve leftovers with a side of scrambled eggs tomorrow; practice getting your veggies in morning, noon, and night.

You might be wondering how much this recipe makes. The answer—well, that depends. There are variables involved with cooking, like the size of the vegetables or eggs you're using. Estimate the mixture to yield between 22 and 24 standard-size muffin cups.

Instead of brushing baking cups with oil, you may use paper liners or a silicone muffin tin.

Don't have a pressure cooker? Prepare your cauliflower the old-fashioned way. Steam for about 20 minutes over a pot of boiling water on the stove.

Feel free to substitute frozen cauliflower florets for this recipe (follow the cooking instructions on the package).

"OPEN SESAME" BAGELS

In college, when I would oversleep and miss the cafeteria breakfast (which happened often), I treated myself to a fresh bagel—hot from the bakery—on the way to class. I can still picture the thick layer of melting cream cheese! As I began to change my eating habits, though, bagels, with around 50 carbs each, were one of the first foods to go. I knew this was a food I would miss. Since bagels are THAT meaningful to me, I designed this A+ copycat recipe.

Serves 10 (1 bagel per serving)
Net carbs: 2g net carbs per serving
Prep time: 5 minutes
Cook time: 17 minutes

1¼ cups shredded whole-milk mozzarella cheese
1 ounce full-fat cream cheese, softened
1 large egg, beaten
¾ cup Carbquik Baking Mix
2 tablespoons sesame seeds

1. Preheat oven to 400°F. Spray a small donut pan with nonstick cooking spray.

2. In a medium microwave-safe bowl, add the mozzarella cheese, cream cheese, and beaten egg. Microwave mixture for 1 minute. Stir, then microwave again for 30 seconds. Fold in Carbquik and blend until dough forms.

3. Divide dough evenly into 10 balls.

4. Poke a hole into the middle of each ball using a finger. Press each ball into donut pan, reforming shape if necessary. (If a donut pan is unavailable, use your hands to form dough into 10 bagel shapes, 2½ inches in diameter, and place on greased 8 x 12-inch nonstick baking sheet.) Sprinkle evenly with sesame seeds.

5. Bake 15 minutes until browned. Remove bagels from oven and serve warm.

Extra Easy Keto Tips & Options

Freeze leftover bagels. Your future self thanks you.

Enjoy your bagel with butter, cream cheese, or both? (It's hard to believe you're losing weight, I know!)

Get creative with the type of bagels you make. Skip sesame seeds and top with a pinch of everything bagel seasoning (store-bought or blend your own). This yummy mix contains equal amounts of poppy seeds, white sesame seeds, black sesame seeds, dried onion flakes, dried garlic flakes, and coarse sea salt.

This recipe presents a perfect opportunity to try a no-sugar-added jam or preserves from the grocery store. Strawberry, raspberry, blackberry, peach, apricot—there's a low-carb flavor for everybody. Would you like to try making your own? I'll teach you how. In a small saucepan, heat 1 cup of strawberries (frozen, whole) and 2 tablespoons of water. Bring to a boil, then reduce heat. Simmer until berries reach desired jam consistency (about 15 to 17 minutes), stirring often. Remove from heat and add 2 tablespoons 0g net carb sweetener and 1 teaspoon unflavored sugar free gelatin powder. Whisk until dissolved. Serve warm or store in the refrigerator for up to 1 week. Jam thickens when cooled.

"I FOUND MY THRILL" BLUEBERRY CHAFFLES

Have you joined the chaffle bandwagon? They're relatively new to the keto community. A chaffle is essentially a cheese waffle (but that sounds clumsy . . . thus, "chaffle"). Whoever thought of pairing such odd ingredients deserves a big hug. Chaffles are ah-mazing! Plus, they're easy as pie to make. Notice the short list of ingredients. A blueberry slant is my personal favorite—it's oh so scrumptious.

Serves 2 (1 chaffle per serving)

Net carbs: 3g net carbs per serving

Prep time: 5 minutes

Cook time: 5 minutes

1 large egg

¾ teaspoon pure vanilla extract

3 (1-gram) packets of 0g net carb sweetener

2 tablespoons almond flour (super-fine, blanched)

½ cup shredded whole-milk mozzarella

1 tablespoon blueberries

1. Spray a large waffle iron with nonstick cooking spray and pre-heat.
2. In a small mixing bowl, whisk egg with vanilla and sweetener. Add almond flour and mozzarella, then stir until blended.
3. Gently fold in berries.
4. Distribute batter evenly among two waffle forms making sure berries are equally divided and spaced out. Close waffle iron and cook 4 to 5 minutes.
5. Use a plastic fork to gently remove chaffles from iron.
6. Divide onto 2 plates and serve warm.

Extra Easy Keto Tips & Options

Be on guard for the ooze factor. Chaffle batter tends to escape the waffle iron when poured too close to the edges.

Blueberries are a delicate bunch. Gently fold them in or risk broken berries (and blue chaffle batter!).

Not a fan of blueberries? *No worries.* Omit this ingredient (and be sure to subtract those net carbs).

Mix it up. Substitute equal amounts of sugar-free chocolate chips or raspberries the next time you make this recipe.

Top your chaffle with even more happiness. Melted butter and sugar-free pancake syrup? *Yes, please.*

MILKSHAKE RATTLE & ROLL

Not everyone has a high-powered blender capable of crushing ice. They don't make them like they used to! For decades, I lugged my dinosaur of a blender around as I moved from house to house. While the pitcher suffered a crack along the side (held together with duct tape, thank you very much), I refused to buy a replacement. That old blender sure was a workhorse for blending up smoothies and shakes. She out-performed them all.

Serves 2 (approximately 12 ounces per serving)

Net carbs: 2g net carbs per serving

Prep time: 5 minutes

1 cup unsweetened almond milk

1 tablespoon heavy whipping cream

3 (1-gram) packets of 0g net carb sweetener

½ teaspoon pure vanilla extract

1 scoop (31 grams) low-carb vanilla protein powder[90]

2 cups ice

¼ teaspoon sugar-free cherry gelatin (from a .3-ounce box)

1. Combine all ingredients except ice and gelatin in a large blender. Add ice gradually and pulse in 30- to 60-second intervals until consistency is blended and creamy.
2. Add gelatin and blend for 30 seconds.
3. Divide between 2 pint glasses and enjoy with a friend.

---

90. Quest or Premier Protein are popular brands of low-carb protein powders.

Extra Easy Keto Tips & Options

If your blender has seen better days, start with crushed ice.

Live on the edge. Try using an unfamiliar flavor of sugar-free gelatin the next time you make this recipe.

Take your dessert to the next level with a short blast of "real deal" canned whipped cream topping. *No joke!* With a mere 1 gram net carb per 2 tablespoon serving, you won't have to lose sleep over the decision. Go ahead and splurge.

BLOOPERS & BOO-BOOS

Reprogramming your brain takes time. There will undoubtedly be some twists and turns throughout your weight loss journey. Don't get frustrated. It doesn't mean you're doing anything innately wrong. Navigating obstacles is part of the process. The art is not letting these throw you off course. Be strong. Feel confident that you can handle whatever comes your way.

> When you have a strong mindset about what you're going to eat, you become unstoppable. This comparison might seem extreme, but it makes me think about people with food allergies. How carefully do you think they monitor the foods they eat? And the preparation? Especially if a reaction could be life-threatening, I'm confident that knowing details about food drives every decision. I realize eating sugar or flour isn't on the same level as this. But it makes me wonder. *What would happen if we applied the same fortitude?*

Sticky situations, screw-ups, they're going to happen. Instead of wallowing in disappointment, get right up, dust yourself off, and get back on the horse. *Giddyap!* Acknowledge and move on.

KETO KING & QUEEN

It's interesting to pick the brains of successful people on DIRTY, LAZY, KETO. No matter the circumstances, they find a way to make it work. I had a long conversation with a husband-and-wife team whose positive attitude and grit really stood out. The couple drove semitrucks for a living, away from their kitchen (and comfort zone) for long stretches. Many people would assume that traveling so much would make healthy eating inconceivable. Not for these two! Being on the road did not stop them from losing weight. *No siree, Bob.* They kept a cooler of low-carb snacks in the cab and chose keto-friendly foods when dining at restaurants (always thinking one step ahead). Impressive.

I cracked up when the husband regaled a struggle from the road. I expected him to complain about a lack of food variety (nope, not a problem). It was finding a tool to poke more holes in his belt (because it still had some life left in it). As he lost weight, his clothes became loose. Drilling more notches—not buying a replacement—seemed like the best wardrobe option (his wife may or may not have disagreed). What a hoot! Aim to be like these admirable road warriors. Seek solutions, not excuses, when faced with adversity.

KETO CONNECTION

Surround yourself with like-minded supporters for encouragement. Feel the momentum of being part of a group: when everyone heads in the same direction, like a school of fish, the energy can help pull you along ("*Just keep swimming.*"). Being around others who can empathize must be a priority. If not in person, then look online.

There are others out there like you; I guarantee it. When I first started, I created a private Facebook group with only my husband and one friend added for support (between you and me, I may have forced them into joining). Then it expanded into so much more. It didn't take long for me to find "my people." I started connecting with hundreds of thousands of low-carb eaters from all over the world.

Whether you link up with my digital community (details provided in Resources) or quietly team up with the gal sitting next to you at work, finding the right support makes the journey much easier. You don't have to go at it alone.

CARRY ON & KETO

Something that continues to amaze me is the impact of celebrating every step toward change (for even the smallest of achievements). Positive feedback is powerful! It inspires us to do more. Don't hold back with self-praise. Make a big deal out of *everything*. I call this the "woot-woot" technique. Say encouraging things to yourself at home (in the mirror) or in public (like on social media). Go ahead! Pat yourself on the back.

Drinking my water here . . . woot-woot!
I finished walking the dog . . . ta-da!
Vegetables are prepped for the week . . . geared for takeoff!

There is nothing wrong with working toward prizes, either (provided they aren't high-carb foods that sabotage you). Working toward a milestone suddenly becomes more motivating when attached to a reward, wouldn't you agree? Don't wait until you reach your "final goal" to get excited. Achieving weight loss breakthroughs, even the early ones, are a BIG deal. Gold stars don't have to cost a lot of money (they can even be free). Include activities that honor your changing shape. Be creative! I'll share some festive examples to get you going.

KUDOS FOR KETO

- Take on a fresh hairstyle or color to showcase the new you.
- Invest in new kitchen items (colorful cutting boards, water bottle, lunch pail).
- Wear shapely boots (that fit over your calves).
- Take a trip to the movie theater (and relish sitting comfortably in the chair).
- Set up a home pedicure station (and paint your toe nails for perhaps the first time in a while).
- Show off your figure with a photo shoot (ask a teen to counsel you about flattering poses and the best camera angles).
- Purchase a new set of bath towels (and treasure how they wrap *allllllllll* around your body).
- Document how you're feeling in a journal entry (also a delight to read again later).
- Wear a swimsuit. Take a plunge!
- Go dancing. Hiking. Ice skating? (Something you couldn't or wouldn't do "before.")

- Take a trip to an amusement park (being able to fit in a ride car feels amazing).
- Try out a new recipe—so many choices inside the *DIRTY, LAZY, KETO* cookbooks.

KETO COUNTDOWN

What waits for you at the end of this journey, for some, will be somewhat of an eye-opener. You'll see impressive changes on the bathroom scale; that's a given. For many, though, the true blessings of DIRTY, LAZY, KETO will have nothing to do with weight loss. Increased energy, confidence, stable moods, pain-free joints, and sharp thinking—these are only the beginning! Your overall health and quality of life will improve.

DLK gives you the whole package.

> Listening to the Bob Marley song "Three Little Birds" (one of my favorites to play on the ukulele) helps put my anxiety in perspective. *"Don't worry about a thing because every little thing is gonna be all right."*

As we prepare to part ways, I want to give you some rock star advice. Rather than stressing about doing things *correctly*, think about doing your *best*. That's all we can really ask of ourselves. Make decisions you feel proud of and then repeat them—that's it!

(Oh, and don't be a Keto Karen.)

Tackle one meal, one snack, one carb at a time.

Have faith in DIRTY, LAZY, KETO . . . and yourself. A bigger life awaits. You are worthy of a healthier and happier existence.

Choose *Extra Easy Keto* and hop off the dieting merry-go-round at last.

Congratulations. You did it! This completes your week of training. A round of applause for the graduate, please. (I'm humming "Pomp and Circumstance" right now.) Throw your hat in the air and do a little happy dance. You got this, my friend. Go forth and keto!

 Day 7 Marching Orders

1. *Time to show off. Plan a week's worth of meals. Bonus points for cooking up at least one meal from "scratch." (If you post pics of your creation on social media, be sure to tag me @ dirtylazyketo so I can cheer you on!)*
2. *Expect mistakes. Describe how you plan to react.*
3. *Gather support to help prod you along (family, friends, online group).*
4. *Document and celebrate incremental successes. Make a BIG deal out of everything!*

Resources

For a free newsletter with support and updates from the author, sign up at www.dirtylazyketo.com.

Get involved in the DIRTY, LAZY, KETO community:

- www.youtube.com/c/DIRTYLAZYKETOStephanieLaska
- www.facebook.com/dirtylazyketo
- www.instagram.com/dirtylazyketo
- www.pinterest.com/dirtylazyketo
- www.twitter.com/140lost

PODCAST

DIRTY, LAZY, KETO Podcast by Stephanie Laska

Acknowledgments

I often receive messages from readers that start with "You'll probably never read this . . ." (before telling me their story). I assure you, I do! There is nothing more rewarding than hearing how DIRTY, LAZY, KETO has impacted your life. I treasure your letters, reviews, messages, and posts. Your heartfelt feedback means the world to me.

We're a family, you and I. Though we may have never met, we share similar secrets and struggles about food. And there are others! Together, we are part of the DIRTY, LAZY, KETO community—a safe place to learn and gain support. Since the beginning, my vision has been to let others know they are not alone.

So many people helped make this dream possible. My husband, "Wild Bill," has been at my side every step. From holding my hand in the green room at NBC's *Today* show to waking up at dawn (every weekend, people!) to edit my writing, his passion and commitment never cease to amaze me. *I appreciate you, Bill!* The DLK entourage also includes our two children, Charlotte and Alex, who (at times begrudgingly) took on unofficial roles as social media advisors, recipe-testers, and (sometimes) dishwashers.

They have shared their childhood (and much of Mom's time) with all things DIRTY, LAZY, KETO. I know it hasn't always been easy. I love you both to pieces.

Thanks to the amazing support of St. Martin's Press, and readers like you, the DLK family continues to grow.

#KetoOn,
Stephanie

Index

affordability, ketogenic diets, 138, 145–50, 168–9

alcohol, xvii, 3, 26, 93–4, 111, 148
  beer, low-carb, 43, 80, 125–7, 158, 163, 186, 197
  as dirty keto food, 161–4
  wine, 11, 34, 80, 122, 124, 162, 197–8

alfalfa sprouts, 52, 54, 56, 83, 100

allulose, 66–8, 171

almonds, 53, 56, 86, 88, 106, 109, 117, 125, 127, 148, 163–4, 194, 217

artificial sweeteners, 61–2, 64–8, 86–7, 120, 161–2, 168, 177–8, 182, 191, 195–6
  side effects of, 170
  types of, 170–1

asparagus, 52–4, 56, 83, 100, 113, 118, 144, 180, 194

aspartame, 171

avocado, 56, 83, 96, 98, 102, 113, 117, 125–6, 144, 155, 169, 184–5, 193–4, 196

bagels, 46–7, 69, 213–5

beef. *See* meat

beer, low-carb, 43, 80, 125–7, 158, 163, 186, 197

before/after photos, 2
  fake, 20–1

bell peppers, 52, 54, 56, 83, 99–100, 117, 142, 152, 192

berries, xviii–xix, 56, 58, 124–5, 152–3, 162, 181, 191–2, 195–6, 215–6
  net carb comparison chart on, 96, 98
  shopping list for, 83, 85, 130, 143–5, 147–8

bread, xxi, 42, 46–7, 173, 179
  keto-labeled, 10, 163, 172
  substitutions, 169, 172, 213–5

breakfast meal ideas, 190–2

breathalyzers, ketone, 21, 24–5

broccoli, 51–4, 56, 83, 100, 113, 143–4, 148, 169, 181, 194
  in meal plans, 117–8, 122, 124

bulk buying, 148

"bulletproof" coffee, 120–1, 178, 191

butter, 56, 80, 101–2, 113, 115, 117–21, 169, 178, 190, 193

cabbage, 51–2, 54, 84, 100

caffeine, 34, 60, 79, 93–4, 129, 132, 150, 153, 163, 173, 177, 182–3, 197

calories, 23, 29, 37, 104, 172
    nutritional overview of, 14, 27–8
    restriction/counting of, xv, xvi, 6, 12,
        31–2, 41, 45, 55, 112
canned foods, 144, 146–7
Can't-Beat-It Beanless Chili, 204–5
carbohydrates
    allowance, daily, 39–42
    biological urge for, 69–71
    camouflaged, 46–8
    as energy source, 13–6, 18, 20, 22–3,
        27–8, 37–8
    fast-burning, 42–4, 46–9
    fat paired with, 51–3, 115
    in meal plans, 112–27
    nutritional overview of, 14, 27–8, 37–8
    Nutrition Fact labels as guide for,
        60–8, 76
    obesity's tie to, 45–6, 76
    portion control and, 44, 57–60, 63,
        97, 184
    restriction of, xvi–xviii, 1, 6, 12–36,
        37–76
    slow-burning, 38, 42–3, 51–7, 76
    tracking/chronicling consumption of,
        71–6, 190
carb tracker worksheets, 74, 190
cauliflower, 51–4, 56, 84, 100, 130, 142,
    145, 152, 160, 162, 180–1, 184,
    211–3
    in meal plans, 113, 117, 119, 121–2, 124
celery, 52–4, 56, 84, 100, 122–3, 125–6,
    150, 152, 185, 194
cereal, 23, 42, 47
    keto, 67–8, 164, 169, 173, 179
chaffles, 173, 180, 215–6
cheese, 16, 34, 49, 53, 56, 58–9, 102, 106,
    152, 161–3, 165, 173, 179–84, 190–3,
    206–8
    in meal plans, 113, 117–26
    shopping list for, 80–2, 130, 142, 147–9
chemical additives, 158, 167–8
chicken. See poultry
Childhood Chicken Nuggets with Honey
    Mustard Dippin' Sauce, 199–200
chocolate, 86–7, 164, 167, 173–4, 176,
    182, 194, 196
    in meal plans, 122, 124–5, 127

coconut, 56, 87–8, 90, 96, 102, 125, 127,
    146, 178, 181, 194
coffee/caffeine, 34, 60, 79, 93–4, 119,
    122–5, 129, 150, 153, 163, 173, 177,
    182–3, 197
    "bulletproof," 120–1, 178, 191
cooking tools, quickie keto, 140
cottage cheese, 43, 47, 56, 81, 106, 124–5,
    192
cravings, xv, 69–71, 75–6
    dirty keto as tool for, 166–7, 185
    tips for, 181–2
cream, xviii–xix, 34, 43, 53, 55–6, 60,
    81–2, 91, 113, 125, 148, 150, 161,
    163, 173, 176–8, 182, 191, 195–6,
    217–8
cream cheese, 102, 148, 194, 213–4
cucumber, 52, 54, 84, 100, 119–20,
    152, 182

dairy, xvi, 14, 27–8, 42–3, 47, 54, 56, 101,
    106. See also specific dairy products
    shopping list for, 80–2
desserts/sweets, 132, 195–7
    cravings for, 167, 185
    in dirty keto, 158, 169, 173, 181–2, 186
    in menu plans, 119–27
    shopping suggestions for, 86–7, 91–2,
        147, 169, 181–2
dinner meal ideas, 192–3
dirty keto foods, xx, 3
    advantages of, 160–1, 177–86
    chemical additives in, 158, 167–8
    convenience of, 159, 160, 185–6
    cost/accessibility of, 168–9
    disadvantages of, 166–76
    as emotional support aid, 180–1
    list of, 161–4
    nutritional value of, 166–7
    substitution of high-carb foods with,
        177–81
    temptation management and, 159–60,
        172–6, 186
    weight loss interruption due to,
        170–2
DIRTY, LAZY, KETO, 43, 187–8. See also
    ketogenic diet "keto"
    DLK Commitment for, 189

Food Pyramid, 42, 54, 56–7
    vs. strict keto, 28–35
drinks, 79–80
    keto-friendly, 197–8

egg(s), xviii, 14, 22, 28, 54, 56, 81–2,
        101–2, 106, 109–10, 113, 130, 142,
        145, 148, 152, 161, 181, 184, 190–1,
        195
    fasts, 10, 33, 35, 165
    in sample menus, 117–20, 125–6
erythritol, 61–2, 65, 68

fasting, 6, 16–7, 132, 151
fat
    diets higher in, xvi, 12–5, 17, 19–20,
        22–3, 30–1, 33, 37, 51–3, 101–2
    diets lower in, xv–xvi, 45, 101, 114
    as energy source, 12–5, 17, 19–20,
        22–3, 28–9
    in meal plans, 112–27
    net carb comparison chart for, 102
    nutritional overview of, 14–5, 27–8
    paired with vegetables, 51–3, 115
FDA, 67
fiber, 14, 28, 37, 43, 51
    increase of, 115–6
    on nutrition labels, 61–2, 64–5, 68
food, keto-friendly, 77, 110–1
    fat-based, 101–2
    fruit-based, 95–8
    grocery list for, 79–92
    keto-labeled brands of, 10, 23, 67–8,
        92–3, 163–4, 169, 172–3, 179
    meal plans with, 78
    protein-based, 102–9
    vegetable-based, 98–101
Food Pyramid, DIRTY, LAZY, KETO,
        42, 54, 57
    diagram, 56
Fortunate Chicken Fettuccine Alfredo,
        202–3
frozen foods, 144–5, 147, 148
fruit, xvi, 14, 18, 20, 28, 43, 54, 95, 97, 115
    berries, xviii–xix, 56, 58, 83, 85, 96, 98,
        130, 143–5, 152–3, 162, 181, 191–2,
        195–6, 215–6
    net carbs comparison for, 96, 98

shopping list for, 83, 85–6, 90
    tropical, 42, 46–7, 56, 96

gelatin, 87, 97, 119, 121, 142, 162, 181,
        195
glucose, blood (blood sugar), 5, 25, 27,
        42–3, 46, 50, 97, 116
    as energy source, 12–3, 15, 19, 38,
        69–70
grains, 14, 28, 45–7. *See also* bread
granola/granola bars, 47, 169, 173
green beans, 52–3, 83–4, 100, 143–6, 160,
        162, 184, 193
    in meal plans, 117, 119, 121

hair loss, 26–7
halitosis, 25, 26
hard candy, 91, 153, 162, 182, 197
health
    keto diet and, 4–6, 50, 222
    obesity's impact on, 45–6, 76
Holla Jalapeño Poppers, 201–2
hydration, 93–5, 111
hydrogenated starch hydrolysates (HSH),
        66

ice cream, xviii, 23, 59, 65, 81, 147, 158,
        163, 169, 171, 173, 176, 179, 182
"I Found My Thrill" Blueberry Chaffles,
        215–6
intermittent fasting (IF), 16–7, 132, 151
isomalt, 65

jalapeño, 54, 84
    poppers, 53, 185, 201–2
Jones, Mike, 22

ketoacidosis, 22–3
keto-branded foods, 10, 23, 67–8, 92–3,
        163–4, 169, 172–3, 179
keto-flu, 10, 94–5, 201
ketogenic diet "keto," xvi, xviii–xxi,
        1–2, 7
    alcohol consumption in, xvii, 3, 11,
        26, 34, 43, 80, 93–4, 111, 122, 124,
        125–7, 148, 158, 161–4, 186, 197–8
    boobie traps in, 9–11
    case studies on, 32–5

ketogenic diet "keto," (*continued*)
    checklist for, 25–6
    comfort food substitutions for, 180–1
    cooking tools supporting, 140
    dirty keto foods as part of, 158–86
    food recommendations for, 77–111
    meal ideas for, 189–98
    myths *vs.* facts about, 17–25
    physiology behind, 11–6, 21–2, 27–8
    routine, development of, as strategy
        for, 139–57
    scam/hoax products for, 10, 20–2, 23
    self-encouragement/reward in, 220–3
    side effects of, 4–6, 25–7, 50, 222
    "strict" *vs.* "DIRTY, LAZY, KETO,"
        28–35
    support network for, 219–20
    versions of, 3, 28–35
ketones, 15, 27–8
ketosis, state of, 17, 19–20, 39
    physiology behind, 11–6, 21–2, 27–8
    testing for, 6, 10, 18, 21–5

lactitol, 66
lactose, 42
lazy keto, 3. *See also* DIRTY, LAZY,
    KETO
leftovers, 145–7, 154
legumes/beans, 14, 28, 47, 204
lettuce, 52, 54, 56, 84–5, 100, 117, 119–21,
    125–6, 129, 142, 150, 168, 192–3,
    195
lunch meal ideas, 192–3

macronutrients. *See also* carbohydrates;
    fat; protein
    balance of, 112, 132
    keto diet's manipulation of, 12–36,
        37, 41
maltitol, 66
mannitol, 66
Mayo Clinic, 114
MCT oil, 32–3, 91, 169, 178
meal delivery services, 10
meal ideas, keto, 189
    beverage, 197–8
    breakfast, 190–2
    dessert, 195–7

    lunch/dinner, 192–3
    snack, 194–5
meal planning, ketogenic diet
    and bad habits, working with, 128–34
    meals ideas for, 117–8
    menu samplings for, 119–27
    and mistakes, troubleshooting, 114–7
    shortcuts for, 129–30
meal plans, 10, 21, 78
meat, xvii–xviii, 14, 16, 28, 53–4, 56,
        58, 77, 101–2, 107, 109, 113,
        143–5, 162–4, 173–4, 180–1. *See also*
        poultry
    in meal plans, 117–26, 190, 192–4
    protein comparison chart for, 103, 105
    recipes with, 204–5, 209–10
    restaurant dishes with, 155
    shopping list for, 82–3, 90–2, 142,
        146–8, 184
    shortcuts for, 129–30
    as snacks, 152
metabolism, 6, 15, 40, 43
milk, 14, 28, 46–7, 177, 180
    plant-based, 80–1, 106, 118, 148, 178,
        191, 196–8, 217–8
Milkshake Rattle & Roll, 217–8
monk fruit, 162, 171
mushrooms, 52–4, 56, 85, 100, 113, 117,
        143–4, 184, 190, 193

net carbs, calculation of, 43, 60–8, 76
No Rules-za Deep Dish Pizza, 209–10
nut(s), 14, 16, 27–8, 43, 49, 54, 56, 58–9,
        86–7, 95, 101–2, 109–10, 117, 163,
        164, 168, 194–5, 206–8, 217. *See also*
        specific nuts
    butter, 34, 53, 65, 91, 107, 125–6, 148,
        152, 161, 173, 182, 184
    in meal plans, 119, 121–3, 125–7
    protein in, 106
    shopping list for, 88, 91, 130, 148
Nutrition Fact labels, 60–8, 76

obesity, 45–6, 76
oils, 27, 102, 113, 148
    MCT, 32–3, 91, 169, 178
    in meal plans, 118, 123–7, 192–3,
        195

nut, 87
vegetable, 14, 87, 163, 169
"Open Sesame" Bagels, 213–5

peanuts, 53, 88, 91, 106–7, 125–6, 152,
    161, 164, 173, 182, 195
pizza, 23, 54, 93, 158, 174, 181, 209–10
plant-based milk, 80–1, 106, 118, 148,
    178, 191, 196–8, 217
popsicles, 63–5, 92, 147
pork. See meat
portion control, 57, 63, 97, 184
    diagram, 58
    in restaurants, 59–60
potatoes, 43, 48, 98–9, 156
    substitutions for, 180, 211–3
poultry, 56, 102, 107, 133, 155, 162–3,
    169, 181. See also meat
    lunch/dinner ideas using, 192–3
    protein comparison chart for, 103, 105
    recipes with, 199–200, 202–3
    restaurant dishes with, 155
    in sample meal plans, 113, 117–9, 121,
        125–6
    shopping list for, 82–3, 90, 129–30,
        142–3, 146, 148, 185
Prize-Winning "Potato" Cups, 211–3
produce shopping, 83–6. See also fruit;
    vegetables
    canned, 144
    frozen, 144–5, 147, 148
protein, 3, 13, 20, 29, 31, 34, 37, 102
    diets high in, xv–xvi
    food comparison charts for, 103, 105–7
    in meal plans, 112–27
    nutritional overview of, 12, 14, 27–8
    powder, 87, 103, 107, 163, 191
    quantity determinations for, 104–9,
        116
    shopping list for, 82–3, 90–2
protein bars, 34, 92, 107, 152, 162, 167,
    169, 182
    sample nutrition label for, 61–3, 65

recipes, Extra Easy Keto, 198–218
restaurant dining, 59–60, 133, 135–6
    tips/recommendations for, 149–50,
        155, 183

routine, development of, 135–7
    affordability as roadblock to, 138,
        145–50, 168–9
    cooking tools supporting, 140
    using off-the-shelf convenience foods,
        142–5
    stress as roadblock to, 138, 150–7
    time constraints as roadblock to,
        138–45

saccharin, 171
sauces, shopping list for, 89–90
seafood, 28, 56, 95, 102, 130, 161–2,
    206–8
    in meal plans, 117–8, 122–3, 125–7,
        192–3
    oily fish, 14, 27
    protein comparison chart for, 103,
        105–6
    restaurant dishes with, 155
    shopping list for, 82–3, 90–1, 143,
        146–8, 184
seeds, 43, 54, 56, 88, 91, 102, 152
shopping
    routine, development of, and, 156
    "shopping the edge" of stores in, 141
    suggested items for, 79–92, 129–30,
        142–8, 184
smoothies/shakes, 47, 54, 97, 147, 182,
    196, 217–8
    protein, 118, 180, 191
snack(s)
    easy ideas for, 194–5
    habits, 132–3
    travel-friendly, 151–3
sour cream, xvii, 56, 77, 82, 102, 193, 195
soy, 147, 153, 155
    milk, 80–1, 106–7, 191, 198
    protein in, 103, 106–7
    shopping list for, 82–3, 87, 89
    tofu, 56, 83, 107, 113, 118
spices, shopping list for, 89–90
spinach, 52–4, 56, 85, 100, 118, 129,
    142–5, 161, 190–1, 206–8
Splenda (sucralose), 161, 171
Splendid Spinach Salad with Salmon,
    Goat Cheese, & Candied Walnuts,
    206–8

Stevia, 86–7, 171
stress, management of, 138, 150,
    156–7
    restaurant dining as tool for, 154–5
    travel snacks as tool for, 151–4
strict keto, 3
    vs. DIRTY, LAZY, KETO, 28–35
sugar. *See also* artificial sweeteners
    alcohols, 43, 61–2, 64–6, 68
    blood (glucose), 5, 12–3, 15, 19, 25, 27,
        38, 42–3, 46, 50, 69–70, 97, 116
    cravings, 167, 181–2, 185
    in foods, 14, 18–20, 28, 37, 42, 46,
        62–8, 75, 95–8
    nutrition labels and, 61–2, 64–8
    substitutes, 61–2, 64–8, 86–7, 120,
        161–2, 168, 170–1, 177, 182,
        195–6

temptation, management of, 159–60,
    172–4, 186
    tips for, 175–6
testing, ketogenic state
    via breathalyzers, 21, 24–5
    via urine strips, 6, 10, 18, 21–5
tomatoes, 54, 56, 84, 86, 96, 98, 100, 144,
    163, 193, 195
    in meal plans, 118, 122–6
tortillas, 48, 92, 153, 155, 162, 169, 172,
    179
tracking system, carbohydrate, 71–3,
    75–6
    worksheets, 74, 190
turkey. *See* poultry

urine strips, 6, 10, 18, 21–5
US Centers for Disease Control and
    Prevention, 45
USDA dietary guidelines, 45–6

vegetables, 6, 14, 28, 42
    dirty-keto, 161–3
    high-carb, 46–9, 98–9
    low-carb, 43, 51–4, 56, 75, 83–6,
        99–101, 113–27, 129–30, 140–8, 163,
        209, 211–3
    in meal plans, 112–27
    net carb comparison chart for, 99–100
    paired with fats, 51–3, 115
    restaurant suggestions for, 155
    shopping list for, 83–6, 142–3, 147–8
    shortcuts for, 129–30

walnuts, 88, 191, 206–8
whipped cream/topping, xviii–xix, 55, 60,
    81–2, 102, 119, 121–2, 125, 148, 150,
    161, 173, 176–7, 182, 191, 195–6,
    217–8
wine, 11, 34, 80, 122, 124, 162, 197–8

xylitol, 65

yogurt, 42–3, 47, 56, 82, 106, 122, 152,
    174, 185, 191, 196

zucchini, 52, 54, 56, 86, 100, 145, 152
    in meal plans, 117, 122–3
    zoodles made with, 53, 130, 179–80,
        192, 202–3

About the Author

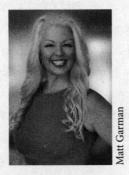

Matt Garman

USA Today-bestselling author and creator of DIRTY, LAZY, KETO, Stephanie Laska doesn't just talk the talk; she *walks the walk*. She is one of the few keto authors who has successfully lost half of her body weight (140 pounds!) and maintained that weight loss for a decade. Her mission is to help as many people as possible fight obesity *one carb at a time*.

Stephanie's honest sass and fresh approach to the keto diet break all the traditional rules of dieting. You might have caught her cooking debut with Al Roker on NBC's *Today* show or seen her on the covers of *Woman's World*. Her story has been celebrated in articles or images shared by *Parade*, Fox News, *U.S. News & World Report*, *New York Post*, *Reader's Digest*, *Yahoo! News*, *First for Women*, *Woman's World*, *Muscle & Fitness: Hers*, *Men's Journal*, *Keto for You*, runDisney, and *Costco Connection*. Stephanie participated in the *USA Today* Storytellers Project and has appeared multiple times on CBS's *GoodDay Sacramento*. She has run a dozen marathons—most notably the New York City Marathon as a sponsored athlete for PowerBar. Not bad for a girl who ran her first mile (as in ever!) at close to age forty.

Want the full story on how you, too, can lose weight for good? Check out the blockbuster *DIRTY, LAZY, KETO (Revised and Expanded): Get Started Losing Weight While Breaking the Rules* (St. Martin's Essentials, 2020), the guidebook that started an international trend to help hundreds of thousands of fans lose weight in a revolutionary new way.

Alongside her coauthor and husband, William Laska (and official taste-testers, children Charlotte and Alex), Stephanie has created a series of support tools: *The DIRTY, LAZY, KETO® 5-Ingredient Cookbook* (Simon & Schuster, 2021), *The DIRTY, LAZY, KETO® No Time to Cook Cookbook* (Simon & Schuster, 2021), *The DIRTY, LAZY, KETO® Dirt Cheap Cookbook* (Simon & Schuster, 2020), *The DIRTY, LAZY, KETO® Cookbook* (Simon & Schuster, 2020), *Keto Diet Restaurant Guide* (2022), and *DIRTY, LAZY, KETO® Fast Food Guide* (2018)—with more to come!

Stephanie also hosts a free podcast, *DIRTY, LAZY, KETO Podcast by Stephanie Laska,* available for watching on the DIRTY, LAZY, KETO YouTube channel or for audio only on Apple Podcasts, Spotify, or wherever you listen to podcasts.

Stephanie and Bill reside in sunny California. When they aren't talking about their third child (DIRTY, LAZY, KETO), the Laskas enjoy bobbing in the ocean, traveling "on the cheap," and shopping at thrift stores.